FIND YOUR
STRENGTH

COLIN SHARP

CONTENTS

To my wife, Eleanor, without whom I could never have hoped to make any sense at all of the humanity I find myself an integral fragment of.

AUTHOR'S NOTE

Despite my all-pervading male, X-generation perspective, I am certain the ideas at the core of my material are applicable to any human body, regardless of sex, age, or body type.

The stories in this book reflect my recollection of the events portrayed. Some names, locations, and identifying characteristics have been changed to protect the privacy of those depicted.

INTRODUCTION

Why I Have Written this Book and What Being Healthy Means to Me

I was not born in optimal health but rather conceived into a body somewhat riddled with defects and into a life that did not innately empower me to find it of my own accord. Yet, despite these challenges—or perhaps because of them—I find the body I am living in as I write this book, at age 40, to be by far the most potently healthy and also most physically broken of anyone else's I have ever known. Moreover, the richness of experience and livelihood that I have sustained because of this excellent physical health has been nothing short of extraordinary.

I say this not to be boastful but rather because the people around me have wondered at it for my entire life, often inquiring as to my *secret*. They see that I am no hyper-focused health nut, that I don't have a gym membership, and that I eat pretty much whatever I want. I only put conscious energy into working out for about 30 minutes every other day. Some have spent time picking my brain in earnest about this, and a few have even asked whether I might be willing to become their personal trainer. Unfortunately, much of a theme as this has been for me, I have somehow continually failed to express the answers in a way that has led anyone down a similar path. I have written this book—a personal compendium of the actions and beliefs that have made me who I am today—in hopes that it may find its way into the hands of anyone whom it may benefit in achieving greater fulfillment for themselves.

Because this book is a retelling of how I have come to act and believe as I do, I present for you the experiences of my life that have shaped these beliefs and behaviors, alongside their accompanying concepts. These experiences are relayed from my perspective, that of a human left to the wilds during early childhood development, then spending the rest of my life learning to integrate into the sectors of civilization through which I have ventured. My eventual education in the biological sciences has contributed strongly to my perspective of the world and of my body.

I would like for the material in this book to impart a sense of biological awareness, in terms of self and in terms of all life other than self. I would also like for this book to encourage its readers to awaken their instincts so they may experience a more fulfilling physical and spiritual existence with the time they have to live. I hope that this book might help to make personal health seem less complicated and daunting, even simple and innate—that it may spur a greater sense of personal responsibility and consciousness with regard to the health of one's body, to the extent that it may even empower some to take complete control over their own healthcare.

Although it contains detailed descriptions of the exercises, techniques, and personal philosophies that have built my body, this book *is not* a workout book. Rather it is a book about how to create and maintain the most potently healthy human body possible, throughout an ever-changing life and within the constraints of our modern environment and the societal parameters that go with it. It is also a book about how to coax fulfillment from this life, through the development of all of the many things that contribute to it. These messages are conveyed through the story of my health and the personal anecdotes surrounding it and, as such, are not intended as a guide or instruction to good health so much as they are an example of someone learning to find their strength.

SECTION 1: THE NATURAL BALANCE OF STAYING HEALTHY

Before I get started, a few words on health itself, for the sake of a shared stepping-off point. The World Health Organization defines health as a state of complete physical, mental, and social well-being and not merely the absence of disease or infirmity.

Being healthy is truly a much more holistic state than our mere physical body being in excellent condition. It encompasses our mental state as well, since our physical body happens not only to house but also to comprise and maintain our minds. Being a highly social species, most of us also require some sense of acceptance from others to feel healthy and good about ourselves. As for disease and infirmity being absent to be healthy, I believe that health exists on a spectrum from dead to the pinnacle of vigor that each individual is capable of, in any given moment, rather than simply a condition that is present or absent. Since no one is born into this optimal physical condition and we all have a built-in complement of microbes and the means to push outside the seams of our bodies, some degree of infirmity will always exist in all of us.

Having an internal population of microbes that increases in diversity from birth means our systems are in a constant state of ebb and flow, forever holding back a tide of impending sickness with inevitably varying success, depending on how strong we feel and how well we are taking care of our bodies. This is why some of us get recurring cold sores or fungal infections in the same places on our bodies for our entire lives, or at least from the time we acquire them.

Examples of pushing beyond the boundaries of our bodies include things like pulled muscles and stretched ligaments, hernias, hemorrhoids, burst blood vessels, and—at the outermost extreme—literally working the body to the point of death. All of these result from forcing our bodies to push harder than is healthy for them, through sheer force of will.

One more aspect to be considered is that of the spirit. This, I feel, has far less to do with what deity we do or do not follow and far more to do with our personal sense of belonging and larger purpose in this grand universe.

With all of that said, it is truly no wonder being healthy is not an easy dynamic equilibrium to maintain and requires a fair amount of conscious focus, as we go through our lives, to upkeep it for any length of time.

CHAPTER 1
The Basic Needs of Our Bodies

I have decided to begin with the basic needs of the physical human body because this is a book about human health and because physical nutrition is a necessary first step in the development and maintenance of everything else.

Whether through instruction or experience, the basic needs of our bodies—air, water, and food—are taught to us at a young age. However, in this modern world of hustle and bustle, we are commonly distracted from these needs, and with a willpower strong enough to ignore the body's urges for them, we sometimes create internal imbalances for ourselves.

Air

Air is our most important need because a lack of it shuts down our bodies faster than a deficit in any of the other needs. Breathing is one of those bodily functions that mostly happens involuntarily but may also be controlled consciously, when we choose it.

When we breathe in, air circulates briefly in our nasal passages, where it is adjusted to the temperature and humidity levels optimal for it to be later absorbed. In our lungs, it passes over the surface of thin, wet membranes with dense capillary beds just under them. These allow fresh oxygen—and whatever else is mixed in the air with it—to permeate directly into our bloodstream, in exchange for spent carbon dioxide (and other metabolic waste), which is then exhaled when we breathe out.

While driving long distances in a warm, vibrating car—staring for hours at the horizon—I subconsciously reduce my breathing rate, until I become aware that white is creeping in around my field of view, a sign that my body is about to lose consciousness. Sometimes I catch myself realizing that I have actually stopped breathing and on a couple of occasions when I haven't, it has led me to unfortunately pass out behind the wheel. Thankfully, these times did not result in any injuries.

A few years back, I helped to coach a young man named Daniel through the minutes between his head-on pickup truck collision with a semitruck at highway speed and the arrival of the life-flight helicopter that was to whisk him away to the nearest large hospital. The look on his astonished face as he came to and admitted to having no memory of what had happened keeps me awake and alert on the road now.

I commonly find myself short on oxygen any time that I sit still without distractions for a lengthy period of time, not just when I am driving. I did not understand why this was such a common occurrence for me until the birth of our second son, Taj. The doctor and nurses had trouble clearing the amniotic fluid from his nose because he had, as they put it, "extremely narrow nasal passages." He looked just like me, all long and skinny in body and face, and it suddenly occurred to me that I, too, had very narrow nasal passages. I often find breathing through my nose alone to be downright laborious and supplement with some mouth-breathing, which I do almost exclusively during exercise.

Oxygen is an absolutely essential fuel and building block for our bodies, which is why our bodies quickly experience dysfunction and then death when denied it. During any kind of strenuous activity, consistent breathing is important for our bodies to metabolize most efficiently and perform at their peak. Depriving our systems of oxygen shuts down the metabolism and other important bodily functions, like thinking. For these same reasons, daily stretching is important, as it increases blood flow to the various tissues of the body, allowing oxygenated blood to replenish the tissues and cleanse them of their metabolic wastes.

When we spend our time breathing in closed quarters, the concentration of oxygen in the air inside of our homes, cars, and offices is gradually being diminished, while its concentration of waste metabolites—like carbon dioxide and methane—increases. Although we frequently open windows or go outside enough to re-normalize these airspaces, the longer we remain inside them without doing so, the less oxygen is available to us in each breath.

Evolutionarily speaking, the human organism is intended to exist primarily outside—where life-sustaining hunting and gathering opportunities exist—taking shelter only when needed to avoid adverse weather, to rest, or to sleep. Finding inside spaces—as modern humans have created them—was possible for primitive humans only in rare circumstances, such as dead-end caves with an opening small enough to be sealed up behind them.

Even our skin has evolved to exist in a fresh-air environment, which is why it secretes oils (to prevent drying out), becomes flushed when we get overheated (to increase evaporative heat loss), and gets goosebumps when we are cold (to reduce blood flow at the surface and raise body hairs for greater insulation) or are feeling threatened (to look bigger, for intimidation effect). Body hair—the adaptive trait tying together all mammals—tends to grow thicker in response to cold weather and thinner in response to warm weather, as any cat or dog owner well knows. This is because the hairs all over our bodies are primarily intended to keep our internal temperature balanced and stable in the face of ever-changing atmospheric conditions outside of our bodies.

Despite a plentitude of research demonstrating extreme human adaptive tolerances to the heat and cold stresses of our planet, for those of us living in modern civilized human environments, living naked outside seems a far-fetched concept. However, consider one example: the aboriginal tribes of the Australian outback, a small subset of contemporary humans. Until their contact with modern humans in the 1700s, they lived out the entirety of their lives naked or nearly so and slept outside, on the bare ground, in temperatures ranging from just under freezing to just over 100 degrees Fahrenheit. This is the most common-knowledge example, and their particular genetic and behavioral adaptations have been well documented, but there are many more like them—including an estimated hundred or so uncontacted tribes worldwide—going on about their perfectly healthy lives, even today.

Fresh, clean outside air is what our bodies are designed to exist in and to process.

Water

Water is our body's next most essential need because it is the solution in which all of our metabolic reactions take place, so if it were to cease flowing in, the body would cease functioning in only a few days.

I hear many people say they do not *need* to drink water because it is already in the other liquids they drink, which is true, in large part. In fact, I have a friend who goes through periods of stress during which he nourishes his body with only Pepsi and cigarettes, for days at a time. His body does not look good during these times, but it carries his soul through it nonetheless.

When we drink a liquid, it is broken up into its simple parts by our saliva and stomach acids before being absorbed into the bloodstream through the intestinal lining. Our kidneys then filter waste products out of the bloodstream, to be excreted through urination or sweat. Therefore, unless we are having extreme bouts of diarrhea or vomiting, nearly every molecule we drink passes through our bloodstream before it exits the body.

This is important to know because, while it is true that all of the other liquids we consume contain some proportion of water, our metabolic reactions require chemically pure water. The more sugars, milk fats, alcohol, caffeine, or other non-water molecules are dissolved in it, the less actual water they are getting, per unit consumed. Since our bodies cannot use Pepsi—or just any other liquid concoction we choose to consume—for their normal metabolic operations, they must perform work to filter the water from it and to groom any unnecessary atoms from these water molecules, until they reach their required purity.

This is akin to losing a bunch of teeth, wherein the body must then work harder, by chewing each bite more times, to achieve a still less efficient result because food particles are not broken up as well going into digestion. This takes the body more energy to process and yields less nourishment from each bite. Common sense tells me that any animal with missing or mangled mouthparts would expect to see a reduction in lifespan compared with its cohorts. Among humans, a decrease in life expectancy has been well correlated with tooth loss, and although I have not found any studies drawing a correlation between early mortality and drinking only fluids other than water, it would come as no surprise to me should it be discovered in the future.

Fresh, relatively clean water is what our bodies are designed to process.

Food

Food is an absolutely essential need of the body because it provides most of the basic building blocks necessary to grow and also the fuel used to power and maintain itself. Cells are the basic building blocks of our bodies and those of all other critters on the planet. Through the process of cellular division, most of the cells making up our bodies produce daughter cells, to succeed themselves, before dying and being broken down for recycling or excretion. Obviously, our hair and fingernail cells are being replaced quite quickly, but researchers have found that nearly the entire body is replaced over an average span of 7 to 10 years. That is, our bodies spend our entire lives perpetually reconstructing themselves from the foods we put in them.

This is why we commonly say "you are what you eat." Like the fluids we intake, solids are dissolved in digestive juices, then further broken down by liver and pancreatic secretions, before being absorbed through the intestinal lining. These components are then distributed throughout the body in the bloodstream for our cells to use for reproduction or as fuel for the body's activities. Anything the body is unable to break down enough to make use of is eliminated through defecation, after the colon reclaims as much water as it can, from remaining digestive juices.

All animals have specialized mouthparts evolved to perfectly complement their specifically intended diets. Moths all have long, straw-like proboscises for extracting nectar from flowers, but each is different and specific to their intended variety or varieties of flower. Like cows (with only cud-chewing molars) and wolves (with only meat-tearing canines), tooth structure dictates the approximate proportion of meat to vegetative nutriment mammalian bodies are intended to consume to balance their fuel and maintenance needs.

Adult humans have 32 teeth, among which only our four canine teeth (eyeteeth) are specifically designed to cut meat. That is, 12.5 percent of our teeth are designed specifically to cut meat. However, the sharper edges of some of our premolars indicate to me that we should have a bit more—somewhere around 20 to 25 percent—of our diet be derived from meat, while the rest should be from plant sources. This is in agreement with the hunter-gatherer lifestyle of our evolutionary past, as grazing on vegetation between successful hunts was the norm and—in my house, anyway—is still reflected from our nightly dinner plates, being mostly plant-derived starch and vegetable with a moderate portion of meat.

Fresh, raw foods of about these proportions are what our bodies were designed to process.

Further Ruminations on Food

Humans have evolved to consume the naturally occurring plant and animal matter of this planet. The further we stray down the rabbit-hole of genetic modification and artificially selecting for size, flavor, or other qualities we prefer in our foods, the more our bodies must adapt to make use of them because they no longer contain the same naturally balanced components. What this means is that—at least here in the United States—our average diets are now further from what was naturally intended for our bodies than they have ever been before, in our entire human history, and only more so every day. Additionally, we have created an assortment of highly processed sugar and grain products that are far removed from anything naturally occurring and also from dairy, which mammalian bodies were not intended to consume beyond infancy. Of course, as we all well know from living this modern life, it is entirely possible for the human body to perpetually reconstruct itself from a plethora of alternative ingredients instead.

Although the natural, unmodified food sources of our ancestral past are still out there—growing in the wild green spaces between and among our scattered bits of civilization—choosing them, like choosing a healthy bran muffin over a delicious cupcake, requires us to have self-discipline. Self-discipline is necessarily intertwined with so many of our important decisions—extending far beyond diet—that it warrants deeper exploration in this discussion of human health.

Self-discipline—the ability to make ourselves do things we know we should, even when we would prefer not to—is something we all struggle with. Over the years, I have developed for myself a mental trick that helps me to choose it, which is structured around time and our perspective on it.

It is true that time stands still for no one. Regardless of what you may choose to do with your present moment, the next moment is always destined to come, and the next and the next. Time never stops marching on, just as it did before we came to be conscious, and just as it will continue to do long after we cease to be. Recognizing this one simple fact is the key to my self-discipline because I know that, so long as I continue to exist, five minutes from now will inevitably come, and so will an hour from now, and so will a year from now. The question is, when this future moment comes, will I look back at the time between my present moment and then with pride and self-respect for what I have accomplished, or will I look back on it with regret for what I have not done, or have not done in a way that would be true to myself?

For example, if I were invited to attend a dawn surf session with my friend, I would know it is something I would want to do, but when the morning comes, dragging myself out of my warm, cozy bed to go paddle out into the cold water in the dark is so very difficult to make myself do. However, as I lie there thinking on it, I realize that if I get to be the me that gets up and goes, I will build my sense of *I can*, be a man of my word to my friend, and get to experience the surreal feeling of catching waves to the rising of the sun. In contrast, choosing to remain in bed means none of that happens, and the me of my near future will most certainly come to look back at the me of this present moment with utter disappointment, not to mention my life will be far less rich for the time in question. I do not like regret, so this always seems to ensure that I do right by myself.

Quantifying the time estimated to do particular jobs helps me with this too, since most of them are relatively quick. I dislike putting away clean laundry, but if I acknowledge that it only takes 10 to 20 minutes of my time and then ask myself whether I would like to come to the end of the next 20 minutes having it already finished or still dreading getting to it at all, my course of action becomes crystal clear.

To continue the discussion of diet, moderation and variation are both important factors to be considered as well. Our bodies are made up of many, many different types of cells, all of which have their own specific cellular components and machinery built into them, so ingesting many different ingredients makes it easier for them to maintain and reproduce themselves. They may be able to do the job—for a time—with only one ingredient (like Pepsi), but they are forced to adapt some creative chemistry to the job, and adverse physiological hiccups are bound to arise.

Relative to the human spectrum, my body has always been high energy, both physically and mentally, so I often find myself chasing activities for stimulation that lead me to calorie deficiency. Volume-wise, I literally eat whatever I want, but I hear my body when it says I have had enough of something because the natural balance of moderation gives room for all of the diversity of diet necessary to build the healthiest body I can.

When I was young, I could just keep eating continually because my metabolism was so high and I was so distractible that I inevitably wandered off to burn more calories before I could even finish consuming the ones in hand. I did not have a real personal reference point for what being *full* meant, as other people did. As I have grown into a middle-aged man, however, I have had to learn to moderate the rate of my caloric intake as the overeating habits of my youth have come to make my body feel uncomfortable. This is an excellent illustration of learning to listen to my body being the key to finding and balancing its optimal health.

As an acknowledgment that our modern lives do not make it easy to maintain an adequately diverse diet, vitamin supplements allow our bodies to get all of the diverse little details they might otherwise become deficient in. I remember my grandmother taking a small handful of vitamin supplements every night with her supper, and my regular vitamin supplement use has increased as my life has progressed. They make good sense to me, so despite my teenage son's insistence that a lack of conclusive clinical evidence regarding the positive effects of vitamin supplements makes them only placebos, I have taken them regularly for many years.

To me, vitamin supplements are representative of the universe around us responding to our expectations, especially the other biota (life) in the universe and most especially the biota of our own bodies. A vitamin is a physical representation of our conscious intent to maintain or change some quality of our body which, when ingested, is literally dispersed throughout and incorporated into our physical being.

Maybe vitamins are just a placebo and maybe they are not, but if I believe they make my body better and that expectation plays itself out, does it really matter one way or the other? I believe that, even if my body breaks down a vitamin I have ingested into more simple components and builds other molecules from every last bit of it—instead of choosing to use any of it for its intended metabolic purpose—the mere ingestion of it alone provides some degree of suggestion to my body.

My personal experiences with particular vitamins have also served to form my strong supporting belief in them. Many times I have tried different supplements that were all reported, among other humans, to be useful in managing the condition I wanted to. In each of these cases, I discovered that one—or at most two—of them affected the desired response from my body and the others did nothing notable. During the more frugal periods of my life, I have also taken every last one of the supplements with no apparent effect on my body, for the sake of not feeling I had wasted my hard-earned money on them. These experiences were consistent in that, if they did not affect the desired change in my body within my first week or two of taking them, then continuing to consume the remainder of the bottle also did nothing for me. This has reinforced my belief in the functionality of the ones that have coaxed their desired responses from my body.

I began taking my first vitamin supplement when I was in my early 20s. My mother, Rachel, was well known for having weak bones and joints that were further exacerbated by the long, skinny bones of her frame providing her with more leverage than was healthy for her joints, and I was born into a similar frame. This genetic preclusion was worsened for me by heavy cadmium and aluminum deposits—inside the old pipes we collected our fresh water from—slowly poisoning the community I came to live in when I was only three months old. As a result, my bones and joints were weakened in their very development, and although it resulted in especially poor circulation when I was young, these conditions have continued to haunt me in a milder form throughout adulthood.

I began having chronically achy and cracking joints as a teenager and went through a slew of possible natural solutions, from *Aloe vera* to turmeric to noni juice, before I fell upon glucosamine. Glucosamine is an amino acid already produced by our bodies, and taking it was just becoming popular at the time. I found that if I took glucosamine regularly, in a couple of weeks my body would stop cracking like crazy and the achiness would subside, and if I stopped taking it, they would return in full force after about a week. I now also take zinc supplements for immunity support and fish oil for the health of my hair, skin, and nails.

I always seek out the lowest possible milligrams per pill because I recognize that, in most cases, natural circumstances in which even that degree of concentration may be foraged for human consumption are either too strong to be palatable or simply do not exist.

I present these ideas about food for informational purposes because they seem to me as biological common sense, even though not a single human I know eats naturally with utmost strictness, myself included. I am completely aware that I ingest *many* things which I know are *not good* for my body, but understanding what my body was *meant* to be sustained by has helped me to buffer it from those unhealthy things and to be internally balanced enough as to remain healthy despite them. Among modern humans, I consider myself very fortunate to have a wife who has always insisted on home-cooked meals from scratch. Although much of her drive to do so stems from the inner satisfaction she receives in expressing her love for us through cooking, I attribute much of our family's good health to it.

Before I dive into the topic of spiritual health, I have a few loose ends to discuss that ride the line between physical and spiritual health, namely sleep, sex, sunshine, and earthing.

Sleep

Sleep is absolutely essential for our mental and physical health, as anyone who has ever had a newborn baby may attest. Just how much each of us needs, however, is highly variable. I know from the experiences of my life that I need about eight hours of sleep every night to feel healthy and mentally stable, and studies have shown that most people need somewhere between seven and nine hours. I can easily go a night or two with less, but I wake up increasingly grumpy with each successive night of reduced sleep. The times I have taken early morn-ing jobs, my overall attitude and feeling about my own health have declined as a function of how long I have endured it. I have always been inclined to be a night owl. Studies are now showing that much of our physical health revolves around good sleep, as the body takes this down time to do a lot of maintenance and repair work that it does not do at any other time.

I fell into a career waiting tables as a means of having both time during the day to play with my little ones and also the money to support them, but now that they are older, I find my evening work schedule still fits the way my body and brain prefer to sleep. Like so many other aspects of personal health, learning to listen to my body's particular sleep preferences and structuring my life around them, whenever possible, has been key in maintaining its optimal performance.

Our bodies, just like those of all of the other critters on our planet, have an internal 24-hour clock, called the circadian rhythm. Among vertebrates, this clock times the release of particular hormones (and neurotransmitters) at particular times of day to keep us on our naturally intended schedule with regard to necessary bodily functions, like sleeping, eating, and bowel movements.

The human clock is based on light levels. When the light gets dim, it induces the production of melatonin to tell us we are tired and should sleep, and when light levels increase, it releases serotonin to tell us we are awake and should be active. This is why getting back to sleep after waking up to use the bathroom is so much more difficult when we turn on a light and also explains the persistent grogginess of graveyard shift workers. It is also an underlying cause of much sleep dysfunction in our modern world, as light pollution and the use of light-emitting electronic screens, especially just before going to bed, have become commonplace. This is something to bear in mind while learning to dial in your body's individual sleep cycle preferences.

Sex

Sex, in my opinion, is extremely underrated as a need in our society. Whether this is because we may choose to live entirely without it—with seemingly no adverse effects—or simply because the condition of getting it or not depends primarily upon personally choosing it in the first place, I do not know.

Like so many of our pre-inclined bodily functions, having sex induces the release of a sequential cascade of hormones and neurotransmitters into our systems, not unlike the process they undergo when we allow our bodies to release waste after forcing them to wait much longer than expected. Sex, including masturbation, releases the body from some degree of tension, frustration, and stress but has also been found to induce strong positive responses in immune function, sleep, and overall health. I believe many of our population's current struggles with anger-based responses, violence, and aggression stem from a baseline of sexual frustration many of us impose upon ourselves in the choice to regularly deprive our systems of this release.

As a human raised without the social influences of other humans, I have always found sex to be a daunting subject because it is so complex and not at all straightforward. Having unmarried parents who separated when I was an infant and did not take on other long-term partners thereafter gave me little example to follow with respect to any of the common human behaviors surrounding sex. By the time I was old enough to have exposure to these behaviors—watching them become suddenly rampant all around me in junior high school—I was already so far behind the curve that I have seemingly been forever stunted, to this day still misconstruing or altogether missing these otherwise universal cues. The mere initiation of this act with another person requires so much inference and immediate calibration as to intimidate me in my daily life, even now.

To add to all of that, the heft of sharing my seed and microbial complement with another person—and all that that implies—has led me to be perplexed by a lifelong hesitancy. At 40 years of age, I have had only four sexual partners in my life and consider the three before my incredible wife to have been high-stakes risks, taken primarily out of the necessity for learning. Of course, I have always been very high energy with respect to sex, as I am in everything, leading me to be all the more confounded by it.

Sex is a complicated and personal issue with a whole lot of variables and individual preferences involved in the process of determining one's particular needs for physiological balance, but learning to listen to the body is a good stepping-off point. For guidance in this realm, I strongly recommend to anyone (be they male, female or otherwise) *The Secrets of Female Sexuality*, by David Shade.

Sunlight

Our bodies were made to be exposed to sunlight, which is why it induces them to produce vitamin D, a nutrient important for bones, blood cells, and immune system function. Vitamin D also assists in the uptake of the necessary minerals calcium and phosphorus. It is because history has made us aware, en masse, that our population tends not to receive enough sunlight (especially in the upper latitudes) that we supplement our milk, orange juice, and breakfast cereals with vitamin D. Conditions of vitamin D deficiency, like rickets and severe asthma in children, were historically far more common prior to this becoming normal practice.

This all follows evolutionarily, as the hunter-gatherer lifestyle of our ancestors could scarcely take place inside, not to mention that our species (*Homo sapiens*) evolved in hot, arid, equatorial Africa and has seen a persistent trend toward reduced body hair. All of our skin—not just our uncovered faces and hands—was evolved to be exposed to sunshine daily, whether directly or through an overcast sky, so it is no wonder we all find ourselves collectively deficient in vitamin D.

Sunlight, as previously mentioned, also induces the release of the neurotransmitter serotonin into our bloodstream. This is the chemical primarily responsible for us feeling awake and alert, but it is also associated with calm focus and an elevation in mood. That is to say, sunlight makes us feel good, which is our body's way of confirming that we are satisfying one of its basic needs.

As anyone who has ever lived in a seasonal location—like here in the Pacific Northwest—may attest, our sleep quality collectively diminishes as the winter sets in. This is because the brighter the daylight we are exposed to, the more serotonin our bodies release, resulting in a more awake feeling, which then induces the production of more melatonin to counteract it when the sun goes down and it is time to go to sleep. When light levels are gradually reduced, in fall and winter, we feel gradually less awake during the day and also less sleepy at night.

From an evolutionary perspective, these are perfectly natural cues, intended to encourage us to hunker down and mostly rest during the winter months—when food resources are naturally scarce—so we do not overexert our bodies without access to the easy calories necessary to replenish. Not sleeping deeply through the winter months also means we are less likely to be caught off guard by any desperately hungry winter predators on their own roving calorie-quests.

Unfortunately, organismal luxuries like just resting in the winter, when the planet gives us signals to, are mostly out of the question in a modern world wherein slowing down means we fall behind, so many of us suffer from seasonal depression that deepens with the season. It is difficult to continue living an active life despite our body making us feel like we do not want to do anything, which is why I tend to work out more and harder through the winter months, to make me feel good and force the release of hormones associated with high activity levels.

The best ways I have found to combat my wife's seasonal depression are to change all of the light bulbs in the house to a higher wattage in the winter and to encourage her to get outside and be active with me during our brief glimpses of sunshine.

Earthing

We discovered earthing about ten years ago when my wife, Eleanor—who is ten years older than I—began having chronic hip pains that bothered her throughout the day but also prevented her from getting good sleep at night. After trying a number of other natural remedies without success, someone to whom I vented frustration about it suggested we try earthing, so I looked it up.

Earthing is the act of touching the surface of the planet, whether with the body directly or via a single path through electrically conductive materials, like wires. The general idea of earthing is that, until just over a hundred years ago, most humans still touched the Earth directly on a more or less daily basis. However, with the advent of rubber-wheeled motor vehicles, rubber-soled shoes, and all the plastics we use to cover our floors, the industrial revolution also ushered in an era of human history in which a large majority of us rarely, if ever, touch the planet's surface directly.

This large-scale change in human behavior also happens to coincide with a dramatic increase of chronic inflammation–related human health conditions, like inflammatory bowel disease, autoimmune disease, psoriasis, atherosclerosis, and others. Chronic inflammation in a body arises because too many of the molecules comprising it are electron deficient, leading them to strip electrons from other molecules to balance themselves. This causes damage and creates imbalance to various tissues, which accumulates into an overall electrical imbalance in the body as a whole.

As the sun's rays come into contact with the Earth each day, they energize the surface particles they touch with light and heat, causing an excitation. This results in excess electrons skipping all over the surface of the planet, making it the largest source of free-flowing electrons in our world that is constantly recharging.

If you have ever experienced a lightening of spirit after gardening or other bare-handed work directly in the dirt or felt the exhilaration of any activity involving your body directly in a natural body of water, then you already know the positive effects of earthing. It invigorates us because it gives our bodies the free electrons they need to balance their own large-scale electrical charge and re-normalizes them to the frequency of the planet, smoothing out their metabolic reactions and allowing them to make more efficient repairs. As with drinking only Pepsi, not having a regular influx of free electrons flowing into the body requires it to do some creative chemical acrobatics to maintain itself and is certain to result in some adverse physiological hiccups over time, like joint inflammations, chronic fatigue, and initiation of the body's various stress responses.

Since Eleanor was aware of her hip pain most when she was least distracted from it—in bed at night—I proposed to her that we try an earthing sheet, intended to flow free electrons to our bodies during the restful healing time of sleep, when they needed them most. Unfortunately, like many, her first response to my suggestion was one of disbelief followed up by some good-natured teasing about my hippie upbringing.

As her condition worsened in the days that followed, I decided to test the theory for us without her knowing by creating my own makeshift earthing sheet using a piece of metal screen (like for your screen door) hidden under our bed sheet, attached by an alligator clip to a wire going out our window. I sanded the paint off a wire coat hanger and attached it to the other side of the wire, driving it into the ground a foot or so from our foundation. The idea here was for our skin to come into direct contact with the screen as a result of the weight of our bodies forcing our skin to bulge through the mesh-like fibers of our bedsheet. Having the window on my side of the bed kept her from noticing the wire for a few days, which was enough for us to experience the positive effects of earthing.

After the first night, she awoke saying her pain was not too bad as compared with the previous couple nights. This was not conclusive enough for me to believe it had worked, so I allowed the experiment to continue for two more nights, after which she awoke reporting that she was feeling great and pain free. I asked if she had noticed something different about our bed, and she promptly felt around under herself and realized I had put the piece of screen under the sheet, right across the part of the bed where our hips were.

I asked her to think back to the last night that the pain had been bad, and she said it was a few nights back, at which point I revealed the details of the entire experiment to her. She was still skeptical, insisting that such a short time being exposed to this new condition could not possibly have produced this result, and it must certainly have been some other subtle change we had inadvertently made instead.

So I removed the screen, and her pains promptly returned the following day, but something else unexpected also happened. When I got up out of bed the next morning, I was remarkably achy, and my joints were cracking like crazy. This, I realized, was my norm at the time, but I was now made more conscious of it because it had been miraculously relieved for the previous few mornings. When I mentioned it to her as we were getting dressed, she agreed that she too had seen a return of all of her *normal* little aches and pains, which she admitted must have previously been masked by the severity of her hip pains.

We immediately plugged in our screen again and ordered a half-sheet from earthing.com, with highly conductive micro-copper wires woven into it and a more efficient rod to put into the Earth. Now, a decade older, we always know when we have somehow come unplugged because we awaken feeling the aches and cricks of our age once more. We consider this our own little fountain of youth and credit much of our youthful lifestyle to it.

As a conclusion to the basic needs of our physical selves, I have a personal account to relay. When I was a young man, I knew another young man who traveled closely within my social circle and with whom I frequently found myself participating in the self-destructive antics of youthful men.

He was always the one in our group who pushed the envelope the furthest, showing nearly no care at all for his physical self, although he was extremely strong in will and in spirit. While downhill skateboarding together, the rest of us would stop short at the top of clearly death-defying drops ending in busy city streets. This man was all about satisfying his spirit, so he went faster, howling maniacally all the way. Many times our adventures ended with him being carried off, bloody and broken, to the emergency room to see if he could be put back together again, but every time he managed to will himself to the front of the line for the next adrenaline rush, just the same.

I was especially amazed with him in that he not only willed his body through so many near-death accidents so often, but he also nourished it almost entirely with alcohol and drugs. He was known to frequently consume nothing else for several days on end, have a few bites of junk food, and then go several more days without. His body was not pretty. In fact, it was gaunt and pale as it could be, but he had a ridiculously rich life, and I witnessed years pass in this way before I moved away.

I heard through the grapevine when he died a couple of years later and was not surprised, but I will forever be in awe of just how far this man was able to push his physical body, beyond what should have been its natural limitations, through sheer power of will. He will always be a reminder to me of just how much extreme imbalance our bodies are able to tolerate at the hands of our spirits before they fail us.

I mention him now only to illustrate that the physical needs of our bodies are somewhat relative to the needs of our spirits and may be widely adapted to the life we want to live.

CHAPTER 2
The Basic Needs of Our Spirits

In contrast to the basic needs of our physical selves, the basic needs of our spirits are not so self-evident. It is rare for a human to learn these needs early in life and our bodies don't necessarily communicate to us when they are not being met. These needs are not so clear-cut as our physical needs, nor are their gratifications and we are each unique in all aspects and degrees regarding them. This makes them much more complicated to satisfy and involves more abstract considerations, in general. My life has led me to an understanding that my spirit has three basic needs: fulfillment, acceptance and living with purpose.

Fulfillment

None of us gets to choose the life we are born into, but we all get to decide what actions we will choose in response to it. In much the same way, as our lives unfold, whatever happens to us is akin to the hand we are dealt, while the way we choose to play out this hand is demonstrated in the choices we make in response to these occurrences.

As much as we would like to believe we *have to do* what we are told to by authority figures, or that we just *can't do* something because of whatever excuses we may contrive, in reality—when it comes to personal choice—there is no such thing as *have to* or *can't,* except in our own minds.

For instance, that a police officer flashes their lights in my rearview mirror does not actually mean I *have to* pull my vehicle over. I could instead choose to make my body keep driving, as if I did not notice, accelerate into a high-speed chase, or even disengage my body entirely, resulting in a collision. Actually, between what we do and how we do it, there exists an infinite number of responses to every event that happens to us, each with its own unique set of consequential outcomes, resulting in a new set of infinite choices. In this way, our lives play out as the intertwined consequence of what happens to us and what we choose to do about it.

The reality of this life is that there are no perfect choices. Rather there is only what we decide to do in every given moment. Finding fulfillment requires an acknowledgment that *all we can do* is to make the best choices we may *think to*—under every particular circumstance in which we find ourselves—because the rest is out of our hands. For this reason, punishing ourselves for making choices we have already made, but that now seem to have been wrong, is absolutely senseless, as there was never any way of knowing the infinity of possible outcomes *when* those choices were made. The universe presented an opportunity to choose, we chose whatever we did, and the universe responded with whatever happened as a result—simple as that.

Every behavioral response to every stimulus is something we each choose, not something we have been forced in some way to do by the universe, by our instincts or by others. That there may be any number of other people or critters or responsibilities relying on us to do as we are *expected* does not change the fact that we must still *choose* to do it in order for it to happen. Having my early family life take place in the wilderness has made me starkly aware that it is even my choice to what extent I live and participate in the human hive. What comes of our entire life is largely of our own choosing, and owning this personal responsibility is the only way I know of to avoid feeling like a victim, with little or no control over my own existence.

The key to finding fulfillment in such a world, for me, has been to learn to manage my expectations, both of myself and of the rest of the universe. I have always liked the Randy Pausch quote "Experience is what you get when you didn't get what you wanted." The point is, when I have expectations that are disappointed, I still have an opportunity to learn from the experience. Experience, coupled with the knowledge I gain over my life, gives me the wisdom to make better and better choices as I grow.

Life is bound to throw me some curveballs, and I am also destined to make some mistakes along the way, so expecting this helps to buffer me from penitence over my unsuccessful actions. The hurdles and challenges presented by this life represent *opportunities* to exercise my built-up sense of self-confidence and prove either what I am made of or just how badly I really want something. Backing down from them is a surefire way to feed that nagging voice in my head telling me I *can't,* and it will lead me down the slippery slope of the fear of failure that ends in me being too frozen with insecurity to attempt anything at all.

Mistakes, though *wrong* by definition, are—in actuality—my most basic and direct natural educator. Mistakes give me negative feedback that results in my feeling averse to doing that same thing again. Without this negative feedback, I would likely continue to burn myself on the hot stove, run out of gas on the way to work, and trip over that same hurdle over and over again, no matter how many times it was presented to me.

How I choose to respond to the negative feedback of my mistakes is up to me, of course. I may choose to curse profusely, depress myself with self-loathing, and go hide away until my ego feels able to carry on again. I may have a hearty laugh at my own expense, pick myself up, and carry on, or I may instead choose any of the other infinities of possible responses.

Like any of the other hurdles or challenges that arise in the course of completing my goals, mistakes represent opportunities for growth and learning. Without them, my life might seem somewhat boring since there would be little struggle to come up against.

Solving my problems and overcoming my hurdles, one at a time throughout life, is akin to the motivational carrot at the end of a string, drawing me on to the next set of hurdles as I surmount one after another. Every hurdle I surpass builds my confidence for the next and teaches me to change and brighten my own world. In stark contrast, every hurdle I decide I *can't* overcome builds my sense that I am an incapable victim of random chance, day in and day out.

For me, a big part of being fulfilled is learning to appreciate everything, even the pain and struggle of my mistakes. I learned to appreciate pain and struggle as a young boy while watching my mother die of uterine cancer. She was not a fan of modern medicine and was already fairly life-hardened when she got sick. At the time, my brother, Dane, and I lived with her in the woods, in the cabin she had built us. Being strong for us was important to her, so she ignored a lot of pain for a long time, before finally relinquishing her body to the medical system.

As soon as she did, however, our lives began to break down while she transitioned into an existence that revolved entirely around treatments and medications. I remember that she was always a strong person—someone the entire community came to for help when serious problems arose—so to prevent us remembering her in any other way, she sent us to live with our father, Bob, in Idaho.

Dane and I watched her die from afar, through letters, phone calls, and one brief visit about five months before she passed. On this visit, we bore witness to what had come of her body, racked with pain and in and out of a wheelchair. Her brain had suffered as well from all the medicine and treatments, and she was no longer the bright sun we spent our childhoods being nurtured by but was instead a nasty, embittered, dark stormcloud of a person. I remember her raving angrily to me—in what turned out to be the last phone conversation we ever had—that they were getting ready to sew up her butthole. I know from what I witnessed that every moment of life she lived—from the day she went to the hospital for help until the day it ended—became incrementally worse for her, physically, mentally, emotionally and spiritually. This experience made me starkly aware that this life may always get worse, until the moment I am not here anymore, so I had better learn early to appreciate everything, even pain and hardship.

Now, when my life seems to be going badly, I begin recounting to myself all the infinite ways I imagine my situation might become worse. If I am having a bad day and it begins pouring rain, I think how grateful I am that it is not freezing rain, or that I am not lost in it, or that I am not dying of hypothermia. If I am enduring the pain of nearly cutting my finger off, I think how grateful I am that it was not cut all the way off, or that it was not my whole hand, arm, leg, or any other of an unending list of worse things it might well have been. This leads me to be suddenly thankful for my legs, my arms, my everything, and the stress of my situation melts away into gratitude for what I do have and where I am in my life. I invariably make better choices with this mindset.

By this same line of thought, that our bodies begin the slow process of deteriorating with age beyond our mid to late twenties means that from then on, the physical tasks of this life will always be easier to accomplish for us in the present moment than they will ever be again, in any future moments—for the rest of our remaining lives.

Through this, I have learned to appreciate everything, in every moment, because worse moments are certain to come and because I do not wish to look back at my life—when I am too old to do the things I would want to—and regret the opportunities that I did not take. Rather, I recognize that the day will inevitably come when I will no longer be able to take the opportunities that present themselves, so I had better embrace them now, while I still have the chance. I appreciate the bad days that come because without them I would not know how deeply I should be appreciating the good days that come. My truly rich existence comes from learning to love life, all of it—good, bad, and otherwise.

When I think of appreciation for every step of life's journey, I always think of having a big mountain to get over. It is easy, almost innate, to appreciate the moment of cresting the peak, even though only half of the hurdle has been surmounted, as the other side must still be traversed. Appreciating the moment of reaching the bottom on the other side is easy to understand as well, since the entire hurdle is now behind me.

However, at this moment that I am finished and looking back at the trip from a place of completion, it becomes easy to understand appreciating the beginning as well—even with the whole journey still looming ahead—because I already know that *I will* get through it. Besides, the beginning always has its perks: my body is fresher than it will be for the remainder of the trek, and my mind yearns to put the miles behind me, leading to a certain eagerness in tempo that makes the time pass quickly.

I think that perhaps the hardest part of the whole experience to appreciate might be just before cresting the peak, when my body is the most stressed from hauling itself uphill against the pull of gravity. Even then, the peak is just right there, providing me the focus of a light at the end of my tunnel and giving me a boost of exhilaration at the thought of impending success. So the hardest part must be the moments just before reaching the bottom of the other side, when I feel the full weariness of the entire journey upon my body without having yet attained the relief of finishing. Still, I have the thrill of a racer approaching the finish line and the lightness of spirit that comes from knowing that most of the job is already behind me. I realize then, of course, how each and every step of the journey should be given the respect of my thoughtfulness and appreciation because not a single one of them exists without the context of each and every other one of them, no matter the ease or the difficulty.

I know that I am never going to be any younger or more resilient than I am right now—for the rest of my life—and I recognize that this is true for *every moment* of *my entire life* as it passes. In the same way, I try to be thankful for the health that I have presently, as though I had just been ill and am feeling the potency of vigor that comes when I finally make a full recovery.

Feeling good about myself is important because feeling positive and feeling negative each produces its own respective cascade of physiological responses, both within my body and outside of it (via hormones and pheromones, respectively). Feeling positive results in the release of several hormones that perpetuate my sense that things are good and also tend to promote good health. Feeling negative results in the release of an alternative set of hormones that perpetuate my sense that things are bad and tend to promote poor health.

Having been a waiter for most of my professional life, I am hyper-aware that how I respond to social stimuli is entirely of my own choosing. If someone does something that upsets me, I could choose to do something I believe may upset them back in retaliation, or I could do nothing at all, allowing them to believe that I have not even perceived their actions. Truly—as with all other situations in life—I have an infinite selection of behavioral responses to choose from, so I have learned to choose ones that serve to make me feel more positive rather than ones that make me feel more negative. This has led me to a greater understanding of self-respect.

Having self-respect is important to finding fulfillment because when I do not respect myself, I allow others to treat me disrespectfully as well, which leads me to feel a diminishing sense of self-worth. Since I get to choose my actions, making choices that empower my self-respect, rather than ones that compromise it, helps to keep conscious that I am, in fact, worth doing good things for. In my experience, without self-respect, self-destructive habits—like choosing disrespecting partners or maintaining abusive friendships—are bound to increase, through subconscious action.

Being a respectable, stand-up kind of human reinforces feeling good about myself, which in turn floods my system with positive-associated hormones and contributes strongly to the good health of my body. Not doing so, on the other hand, reflects negatively on me, which results in negative-associated hormones being secreted into my bloodstream, reinforcing the sense that I am not good and contributing to the reduced health of my body.

Maintaining self-respect requires that I be of my word, no matter what happens in my life. My word is my bond, so if I say I am going to do something, I am most certainly *going* to do it. This also encourages others to respect me because they know that I can be counted on, at all costs. I use this as a tool to make myself do things that I know I should but do not want to do, since all I have to do to commit myself to doing it is to say to anyone that *I am going to*.

I used this trick to make myself write this book, by telling my family members that I would do it. Saying what I am going to do is a way of keeping my particular goals conscious and out on the table, so that I make sure to get them done.

Achieving both short-term and long-term goals on a regular basis is also necessary to feeling fulfilled in this life, as it helps to build up and maintain my self-confidence. This may start with something as simple as a goal to do as many push-ups as I am able to do today or to remember to call my brother on his birthday. Both are opportunities to prove to myself what I am worth, and completing them will result in my feeling better about myself, while saying I will do them but not doing them will result in my feeling worse about myself. Given the choice, I prefer to make myself feel good by saying what I will do and then seeing it through, by doing what I say I will.

Before I move on to the topic of acceptance, I have one more little mental trick to share, which I use to keep myself appreciative of all of the opportunities that come my way. When I have something I know I should do—regardless of whether I perceive it to be positive or negative—telling myself *I get to* instead of *I have to* helps me to keep conscious that every chance I am presented with to do something in this life is an opportunity and not an obligation.

For instance, although at first glance there may seem nothing positive about getting a flat tire on my way to work, telling myself that "I *have to* change this tire to get myself to work" forces me to focus on the obligation of the task at hand and leads me harbor some bitterness toward the universe for having put this hurdle in my way. On the other hand, telling myself that "I *get to* change a flat tire if *I want* to get myself to work" serves to remind me that I still get to choose whether I do this thing or not and that there are actually an infinite number of less-favorable tasks that I could be facing in this moment—or, even worse, I could be somewhere entirely unstimulating, with no opportunities at all laid out before me. Now I am thankful for this opportunity to show how efficiently I may change a tire on my way to work, and my life is more interesting for having had the experience.

I learned this technique because, after our mother Rachel died, my brother Dane and I lived a bland life with our single father for several years, under a veil of depression that had us both paralyzed and numb to the stimuli of life. We hardly spoke or engaged with one another or with the world around us, seemingly unable even to acknowledge the opportunities constantly flowing by. This made life rather unstimulating, and my mental and emotional shell was so very thick that those around me rarely received any response to their proddings and pickings even when they did try to break through, which taught me an important lesson. No matter how hard they may try, no one else makes me do anything. Rather, I choose whether to respond to the stimuli of my life and to what extent.

During this time, I recognized that all of the other kids at school were engaged in any number of activities—some fun, and some not. I began to envy them for all of the brightness in their worlds, which contrasted so harshly with the colorlessness of my own. I realized that even the worst experience I might witness someone around me having was still a whole lot more stimulating than anything I had done for a very long time.

I broke myself out of this depression—of my own volition—by discovering *work*, through which I was immersed in brighter environments and earned the means to take the opportunities that came my way. I threw myself at it head-long, taking every bit of work I could and even spending my free time scouting for more because it kept me out in the bright world rather than in our dark, depression-stifled home. I did not *have to* go to work out of obligation, I *got to* go to work as a means of escape from a less pleasant alternative.

Our father, Bob, had taught us to work hard for him in his one-man (and two young boys) landscaping company from the time I was seven, so I learned to apply that knowhow and work ethic to raking up the neighborhood's leaves for income in the fall, which led to other random jobs throughout the year.

At nine, our older sister, Stacey, took first Dane and then me under her wing at her job. We sold candy and novelty items door-to-door with a vanload of other uncared-for children, under the command of exactly the vagabond sort of characters you might expect to be exploiting cute little kids for an 80 percent cut and paying them no hourly wage. Regardless, we were an adorable bunch, so on good weekends I might chance to clear $120. Summers, I opted to work as many days as I could and began saving for the resurrection of Rachel's old van.

When I was 12, an older friend snuck me into a motel job, fudging the numbers on my hire documents since I was not yet legally old enough to work there. I worked in laundry until I was bored into accepting a position cleaning rooms and then became the property utility man before moving across the street to a Holiday Inn, where their restaurant offered me more opportunities for experience. There I washed dishes, then bused tables and delivered room service, eventually accepting graveyard kitchen-cleaning shifts in addition to whatever daytime shifts I could lay claim to. I became a full-blown workaholic by age 14, juggling school as an afterthought.

I have accomplished far more arduous undertakings since then, but I still recognize them all, no matter how seemingly undesirable, for the opportunities that they are, and I would still rather be doing any of them than nothing at all.

Fulfillment is not tangible, so attaining it sometimes feels like grasping at straws because it is hard to understand the feeling when we are busy—in the here and now—completing tasks and solving the unending problems of our lives. However, looking back at the end of a day, a week, or a year, it is easy to perceive the difference between a fulfilled life and one that is not.

Acceptance

As a highly social species, we humans are affected strongly by the acceptance, or lack thereof, of our families, peers, and social groups. An environment of acceptance fosters the growth of self-worth, while an environment without it leaves us wondering what may be wrong with us and may even provoke us to behave in far different ways than we are inclined, in hopes of gaining acceptance.

That is why Eleanor often points out to me how much we are all, to some degree, products of the environment we choose to exist in because we all tend to pine for acceptance—even if it means doing as everyone else around us is doing, when that is not what we ourselves would want to do. Ultimately, this leads to idiosyncratic regional behaviors shared by entire populations. It also leads me to wonder what each of us might do and be, were we less concerned with what others thought of us.

Having been raised in the woods, away from civilization, for my first five developmental years, learning to find human acceptance has always been a bit of an uphill struggle for me. *Maintaining* any level of acceptance within a given group of humans still tends to evade me, as what is socially and legally acceptable shifts constantly, both from region to region and as time goes by. Legality, after all, has never been defined by morality but rather is an indicator of what is socially acceptable in a particular time and place.

"Hippie," like many trends in human behavior, is an idea that has many facets and degrees to it. Some humans who follow the idea do so only in their fashion sense, while others go further, incorporating its ideals into their everyday lives, through diet and behavior. My parents took it to the extreme, separating themselves from the rest of the human world and taking their family to the trail to live a more bohemian life altogether.

I was conceived on the trail, while my parents traversed the Rocky Mountains on foot with my older sister Serrafina (age five), Dane (just over a year old), the family dog and a mule to carry all of their belongings. Although my brother had just been born on the couch at home about a year prior, when Rachel got pregnant again, they decided it would be best to make their way to a hospital for my birth rather than chancing such an event to the elements, out on the trail.

The nearest place to them that had both a hospital and close friends nearby who could help them was Boise, Idaho. Their friends let us use their school bus, which had been converted into a camper, so my birth certificate reflects our address as the truck stop where they parked it during the time of my birth and Rachel's recovery.

My parents were not married, nor did they feel the closeness of marriage in their relationship, so when the dust settled, they made an arrangement. She took us kids to live with her in Washington State, near her family, while he worked out his situation there in the mountains outside of Boise.

Bob laid claim to a gold mine in the area and proceeded to live off his scant gold pannings in an old Sioux-style teepee he had acquired. Rachel saddled up with some old friends on Cultus Mountain—outside of Clear Lake, Washington—moving us into an old trailer in their front yard while she worked out a longer-term solution.

I call my parents by their first names because we always did, from the time we were old enough to call them. Rachel insisted on it, as a conscious acknowledgment for all of us that she was the *person that she was* and not to be pigeonholed by identifying as the word symbolizing her role in the family. We called Bob by his name only because he was indifferent and we had naturally carried over the idea from Rachel that our parents were denoted by their names.

Dane and I have two older half-sisters, who were each the product of our parents' previous partners and are both about six years older than I. Serra—our sister from Rachel's side—was with us at the time but then went to live with her father for a few years, to relieve some pressure.

Rachel, though sweet enough to us boys when she had attention to give, was known to be quite masculine. She cut trees to clear a building site and a quarter-mile trail to it before building us a two-story house—by herself—from the remnants of a huge barn some neighbors let her de-construct for materials. She felled trees for our firewood every year and could often be found working on her 1961 Ford van (which I later inherited, as my first car) or being called away to this neighbor's or that for help with their mechanicking or some other laborious task.

Dane and I were left to our own devices, more or less raising ourselves on the trails of the surrounding woods, with our two black labs—Bonnie and Bear—as our guardians. Unfortunately, my brother's inner Taurus shone angrily bright when he was a boy, and so, as his annoying little brother, I was left to find acceptance from the wildlife around us—which I did.

Although the deer, birds, and frogs of our woods were rightly furtive around other humans, they seemed to know that I—a small, innocent child, often wandering off alone—was of no real threat to them. Every day I made the rounds through my countless animal friends and felt that they truly accepted me, as much as they did all of their other woodland neighbors.

Our home trail continued through the front yard, separating the house from the outhouse before meandering off through the woods to the powerline trail that acted as a local wildlife corridor. I often found myself waiting anxiously for the local coyote pack to finish filing back through the yard—in the bleak light of dawn—before creeping to the outhouse to do my morning business, unbeknownst to the rest of my family. I suspect Rachel knew what was happening because she would sometimes find me—later in the morning when she got up—asleep in funny positions on the couch overlooking the window to the yard, having fallen asleep while waiting.

When I did make it to the outhouse and finished my business, I would often wander the yard and surrounding woods while waiting for the rest of the house to awaken. I discovered that all of my critter friends had also been waiting for the nocturnal predators to clear out before venturing out for their own morning business. I recognized that we shared many natural tendencies, and I felt a close sense of kinship to them.

This time and place in my life has forever since felt like the home of my soul, where the true me first gained acceptance in this grand universe. It was a golden time in my life, and because of it, the long journey ahead—toward eventual human acceptance—was forever framed from this vantage point. I am Colin, accepted first as a critter of the Earth among the other critters of the Earth. My humanity has always come second to this first, foundational nugget of self, and my perspective on civilization, other humans, and my experiences in the human world has forever since been framed from the perspective of an outsider, looking in. I see humanity in the same way that I perceive every other highly social species on the planet, as intriguing and kind of awesome for all of its intricacy and intensely evolutionarily derived convolutions. However, I can still say—even after all these years—that I feel a less conditional degree of acceptance from most random critters I encounter than from the vast majority of humans I interact with every day. Thankfully, the truth remains that I alone choose the degree to which I do or do not care what other humans think of me or of my actions.

Because we humans thrive, in part, on social acceptance, I have also observed a strong mental tendency toward inclusive/exclusive behaviors among us. Any inclusive group of humans, by definition, excludes all others, leading to an *us versus them* mentality. So long as we choose to accept only certain others, we also choose not to accept everyone else. Whether the group termed *us* includes humans of a particular region, background, belief system, political party, or any other defining characteristic, it also automatically confers a label of *them* to all others. This tendency is so common that it has led to the conception of words like *ethnocentric* (culturally exclusive), *anthropocentric* (exclusive of everything not human), and *self-centered* (in which everything outside of *I* is deemed to be *them*). It also seems to me the reason that we as a species experience so much strife and war. I like to think of acceptance through the lens of the Golden Rule, which is to say that if we wish to be unconditionally accepted by others, then we should strive to unconditionally accept those around us.

Among the other critters of the world, the only natural analogy to this I have witnessed is that of predator/prey interactions, but because hunting is outlawed within dense human populations, most of the Earth's other creatures do not impose this expectation on the average human. That is, the other critters mostly accept us, while we humans generally only choose to accept the very few among them that will conform to our conditions, which we call *pets* and count among our possessions.

Being the only full siblings in the family, our parents decided that Dane and I should remain together but continued to shuttle us back and forth between her (in the woods of Washington) and him (on the gold claim in Idaho) until he moved to Boise, when I was four. With the exception of a short time spent in a Montessori school in Boise that Bob did some work for, I experienced my first real taste of the systematized human world at age five: kindergarten in the small town of Clear Lake.

I remember the start of class on my first day of kindergarten, when we were instructed to line up and take turns writing our initials on the chalkboard at the front of the classroom. My first question to the kid in front of me was, "What are initials?" In annoyance, the boy attempted to explain it to me, but since I had no idea what letters were, or the alphabet, or even my last name, this proved to be the first step in a long school career of social embarrassment. I soon learned to be quiet and not to draw attention to myself, lest anyone become aware that I was actually a mostly feral critter sitting here among them and not a little boy at all, having to be subjected to these complicated little-boy expectations.

One day, toward the end of the school year, Rachel came to pick me up after class, and the teacher approached her, requesting that she go and speak with the office about something. There, they informed her that, while all of the other little boys and girls in my class lined up nicely at the door to sing the alphabet before release every day, I still struggled with the lining-up process and only pretended to know the alphabet, chanting random letters to the pitch and tune of the class right from the very first letter. When asked if she might please do a little work with me on it at home, Rachel snapped back, defensively— something about, if they cared so much what I learned then why weren't *they* teaching it to me—before storming out, with me in hand.

Bob was determined to get his master's degree in Boise, so when Rachel came to terms with her illness a year later, Dane and I moved back with him and were enrolled in a big-city elementary school. There we proceeded to learn the ways of other humans, including all of the complex social dances they require for one to gain their acceptance.

I did not do well, to say the least. My lack of any of the basic knowledge all the other kids had left them to presume that I must be stupid, and with only a vague semblance of the verbal skills they had, I could not figure out how to change their perceptions of me. To add to my lack of understanding, I had very poor eyesight, not being able to see clearly beyond about eight inches in front of my face. Unfortunately, because I was silent and generally successful in my attempts to go unnoticed, no one realized this—least of all me.

I had already been outcast, which only got worse when Rachel died the following year and our household depression sunk in. My peers ridiculed me relentlessly, picking on me in groups and spitting on me from their buses as I walked home in silence, with my head down. Although I still felt the inner security of knowing that nature had accepted me among the other critters, I did not dare even to imagine what it must feel like to have acceptance from other humans.

When I was 13, my math instructor figured out I could not see, and I got glasses. Until that day, I had no idea what facial features or body language *were*, much less what they *meant*, and my clumsy reputation faded away as I could finally see where I was going. I began to understand how to gain acceptance from my peers and set to work building up my own sense of self-worth.

Although I gained momentum in this, I continued to find that humans made generally fickle friends, only liking me at their own convenience and otherwise just as happy to put me down to feel better about themselves or to elevate their own social status. Despite the few accepting gems I found among them, I learned to keep few friends and to have a healthy distrust of humans in general, for the sake of self-preservation.

As a hard-headed baby boomer whose life evolved from that of a nomadic hippie in the wilderness to a master's degree–holding hive-builder as our childhoods played out, Bob's version of caring for his children entailed teaching us to fend for ourselves as soon as possible so that he could be relieved of the additional responsibility. As the youngest, I was a proficient couch-surfer by age 12 and wandered completely away from home—to become a full-fledged street rat—long before high school graduation.

At 19, I met Eleanor, and although she had a lot of work to do in grooming me into a socially and hygienically functional human, I discovered in her true acceptance. I began to have pride in myself and to know the amplification of self-worth that comes from being valued by others, something I hadn't dared to hope for until it happened. My life finally took off.

Having someone who knew, understood, and cared for me gave me reason to care for myself more than I ever had before. I began to value being clean, reliable, and behaving appropriately at the appropriate time and place, if only for her. She taught me, one day at a time, how to gain acceptance in the human world, and learning it from her opened up opportunities for us that I could never have conceived.

When she got pregnant with our first son, Zakai, we had many heavy discussions about how we were to raise him, since we had both received a degree of conditional love from our families growing up that had led us to become uncared-for street kids. We agreed that unconditional love should be the umbrella under which we would foster our child's development, to ensure that he would not have to find acceptance on his own, as we had. Unconditional love means that your expression of love toward someone is not contingent on their behavior. That is, after every conflict with our children comes to a resolution—be it a toddler slap in the face or a battle over teenage boundaries—our bottom line, end-of-the-day message is that we still love and accept them, and we always will.

We knew, from our own experiences, that when family showed us love only if we behaved in a manner that met with their approval, the clear message we received was that love is not a given but rather is earned through a willingness to yield to their control. That is to say, because their expressions of love were contingent upon our behaving as they would have us do, we felt as though they did not truly accept us for who we were naturally inclined to be. We all must make mistakes to learn in this life, but if the acceptance of our family depends on our not making mistakes—by their determination of it—then we are persistently made to feel incompetent in doing what *we* think we should. It is a setup for us to lose our self-esteem, and by adulthood, it is no wonder so many of us struggle to discover who we *truly* are.

That is, however, exactly what needs to happen, because being sincerely loved and accepted requires that we must first know who we are and be consistently true to ourselves. Otherwise, the person attempting to love and accept us is being misled by our own subconscious, just as we ourselves are. I have done my best to come to terms with myself and to learn to be honest with myself about many things that have been uncomfortable or unpleasant to admit, and to resolve them, if only through a lifetime of conscious effort.

My father's example growing up taught me to sweep under the rug any of my uncomfortable actions or words by making excuses and generally avoiding further discussion about them. When I got together with Eleanor, this aversion to taking personal responsibility for my mistaken actions became a recurring theme because I was truly unaware of it.

Since we mostly forget our most formative first few years once they have passed, we all have funny subconscious behaviors we unknowingly exhibit, given particular stimuli, that stem from the example we were shown during that time. When faced with the reality of these behaviors, our response is often denial because we are not actually aware of what we are doing. Acknowledging and changing it requires a willingness to suffer a temporary hit to our self-esteem, as we must admit to ourselves that what we *have been doing* was not copacetic to others.

This one incongruity in my personality nearly busted our coupling early on, and had my sweet wife not had the patience to point it out to me over and over again—while I had the fortitude and humility to come to terms with and change it—we certainly would not have experienced the richness our relationship has provided our lives for the last 20-plus years.

No human is perfect, which is why we commonly repeat to one another the Alexander Pope quote, "to err *is* human..." Having the strength and humility to acknowledge our own humanity gives us the means to work through it, rather than wallowing stagnantly in our own unyielding hard-headedness for the precious time we have to live.

Learning myself and being honest with myself about who I am and what I do is preliminary to being truly loved and accepted by anyone else. I know socially successful people who are very lonely inside—despite outwardly happy marriages and children—who feel generally above reproach and who also fail to find acceptance among even their own close family members. I also know socially apathetic people who find all the acceptance they need in the critters around them, to which they persistently admit all of their faults.

Having respect for myself is preliminary to loving and accepting myself just as knowing myself is preliminary to others loving and accepting me. If I persistently behave in ways that compromise my own integrity—like lying, stealing, not being true to my word or treating others disrespectfully—having respect for myself is not possible because I will be consistently faced with the negative feedback of others' responses. There will be an obvious conflict between the inner me that I perceive myself to be, and the me that is being presented outwardly to others.

Participating in a social group that requires me to compromise my own belief platform to gain acceptance makes me a product of that environment to a greater extent. I try only to participate in social groups that value my unique differences and in which I may be true to myself, although I have learned to show myself slowly when introduced to any new group of humans. I have further learned that my innermost thoughts and feelings tend to be very different from those of the average human, so to avoid inciting exclusive or mob mentality–like behavior, I rarely voice them, and when I do it is only within intimate groups of particularly open-minded and accepting humans.

Respect is earned—even respect for self—by having the strength and humility to admit and overturn the negative subconscious tendencies we have and to have the self-discipline to behave outwardly in a manner that is consistent with who we are inside. For assistance in discovering ourselves, I recommend *The Life You Were Born to Live*, by Dan Millman, as a stepping-off point.

For me, self-respect is a core value, and without it I do not know how one would go about gaining the degree of human acceptance necessary to lead a rich and fulfilled human life.

Living with Purpose

I have been fascinated by animal behavior for as long as I can remember, and human behavior is no exception—which makes sense as we are, of course, animals too. According to science, regardless of whether it is a plant or an animal, every single behavior every critter exhibits (yes, plants behave, too) is the consequence of an interplay among two intertwining forces. The first includes the mechanistic variables of genetic code and physical construction, providing the full range of conceivable behavioral responses. The second are the long-term evolutionary drivers (instincts) contributing to the reproductive success of the species and the whole equation is complicated by the experiential learning of each individual.

As a simple example, mate-guarding is a common animal behavior shared by primates (including humans), lizards, birds, insects, and fish. It is the male practice of standing guard over a female just after copulation. It may range from as casual an expression as merely keeping her attention occupied to literally sealing up her genitalia with various secretions or even—in some of the more unusual species—the breaking off of male genitalia to block the passageway. The reason this behavior has developed in all of these many diverse families is the same: to improve the odds his sperm will not have to compete with those of other males for her eggs. However, the particular strategies employed by each type of critter depend on the mechanisms their bodies possess, the bank of instinctive behaviors with which they have been genetically programmed, and any experientially learned strategies they may have picked up along the way. Of course, humans, with all of our brain power, most effectively employ tactics to occupy her attention in hopes she will not notice anyone else. Regardless, in each case, the instinct *to do it* has carried through the generations of all of these different family lineages because it has contributed directly to the reproductive success of each species.

This is the lens through which all other animal behavior is studied scientifically, although human behavior—being its own complicated beast—has spawned its own field of psychology. Psychologists seek to understand human actions, thoughts, and feelings through analysis of the various biological factors, social pressures and environmental stimuli attributed to them, further applying what they learn to a broad assortment of other human sectors.

In going to college for biology, I discovered that I am more of a naturalist at heart than a biologist. Although both fields study life, the fundamental difference between the two revolves around a difference in core belief.

A naturalist believes observing and studying the life around us is best done in context. This is because life behaves far differently when it is removed from the environment in which it naturally occurs or if that environment sees a sudden dramatic change, like being enclosed. In fact, I find that life often behaves differently than it otherwise would have just for having been *observed* by humans, even *in* its context. Not one single life form on planet Earth exists in isolation; all of them are part of an intricate web of interaction that includes—in one subtle way or another—every other life form on the planet.

Biologists, on the other hand, believe life is best studied by compartmentalizing it into controlled environments of their own design, which streamline behavioral responses to give them what they perceive to be cleaner data, with fewer *irrelevant* variables to cloud interpretation. In my observation, the shock organisms undergo through this process induces thoroughly unnatural behavioral responses to whatever stimulus is applied because they are no longer comfortable to do as they are inclined. I cannot deny that the evidence gained through the common biological practice of removing physical critter mechanisms—with subsequent testing under various laboratory conditions—is quite compelling and has led to many amazing further discoveries. However, to me, this practice is like the many other things that humans have been so excited to learn they could do that they never paused to question whether it was ethical or respectful to do so before going ahead and doing it. I feel that humans have justified this inhumane treatment of our distant relatives because, of course, among humans, human life is valued far more than any other form of life.

I've often wondered about my wife's drive to save every tragic teen she comes into contact with, as a result of her own life's experience. I asked her about it once, and she said it was like the story I told her of my brother and me, as children on the beach, rushing to scoop up and toss back the countless jellyfish that were beached by the tide. She pointed out that our desire to change our world was not made irrelevant by the fact that we could not save them *all* because we were making the difference we craved in the lives of *each and every one* that we did save.

I consider all life to be precious—no matter how seemingly insignificant—perhaps because I relate to the underdogs of this world, having felt insignificant myself for much of my own development. Severely irritating as I may find an insect flying around my head to be, I think *that* alone is by no means sufficient justification for ending its life and any future contributions it may otherwise make to the life that exists after our encounter. To me, the countless research subjects of human experimentation are victims of humanity's lust for knowledge, and I find myself pondering what their fates must be like from their perspectives. I sense a little sigh of relief from every tiny insignificant-seeming bug and spider that I pass by once I am gone and they have not been inadvertently crushed under my enormous feet. I know that they are in some way thankful to still *be*, and I feel a little sense of relief myself for not having casually ended them. I try to be as conscious as possible to treat with care all of the life that I exist in the context of, out of great respect and thankfulness for my own life.

For these reasons, my study of animal behavior—be it human or otherwise—tends to be purely observation-based, with the least possible amount of subject interaction involved. Although I have learned a lot about human behavior from my own various human relationships, my "outsider looking in" perspective and ease in going unnoticed have amplified my observational learning of the subject. Through observation, I have learned that the most common human behavioral hindrance to living a life with purpose is *carelessness*.

Carelessness is a learned human behavior. I have seen it learned through the careless example of others or from families or other social groups, wherein negative criticism or negligence is the teaching technique primarily employed by those in authority. When an individual consistently receives negative feedback—or no response at all—to their actions, over time they begin to feel that what they do does not matter, since good, mediocre, and poor performance are all treated the same. This leads to a feeling of general worthlessness and insignificance as well as an overall apathy toward the entire rest of the world.

It takes only two humans to do this dance, but once it is ingrained, it quickly spreads—much like a disease—to others in their community, who observe that their indifference does not lose them their place in society. For a while, those who take care in their actions continue to do so, but as time passes, they gradually become less careful because there is no incentive for caring, as they are receiving equal credit or pay to those who do not care. It becomes a subtle competition to see who can care the least without suffering adverse effects. Since conflict is uncomfortable and therefore generally avoided in human social environments, so long as this carelessness is not too overt, no one raises a red flag, and the attitude persists or increases. Unfortunately, as we are now a global hive of billions, carelessness is simply not sustainable for us anymore as a species.

Were all the world's humans to be collectively careless about important things like self and others, our use of the resources that support all the critters of the planet and where and how we dispose of our many waste materials, then war, disease, and famine—nature's normal population control measures— would quickly reduce our population until it was small enough to be carefully sustained. In this way, how many humans care about their lives, and to what degree, determines how many we may support with our hive's given knowledge and resources at a given time. It also determines, as a consequence, how many of the other critters the planet has room and sustenance for as well. It is because so many *do* care about these things that we have come to learn our way out of these natural controls through things like peace rallies, vaccines, and hunger drives.

However, our ability to overcome these natural processes have allowed us to come to our current state, in which there are so many humans on the planet as to have destabilized our natural balance relative to the populations of the other critters. Like all predators, we exist at the expense of those we consume, and since we are such diet generalists as to require a wide variety of other organisms for sustenance, as a species we have now consumed our way through a vastly disproportionate share of the life around us. Each of us bears some small percentage of this biological burden in the number of calories required to see us through our lives, our carbon footprint, and how much material goods we acquire and dispose of in our lifetime.

As individuals, try as we might, there is unfortunately no way to reduce our piece of this burden to nothing. We may only do the best we can with what we get, one day at a time. Unfortunately, knowing these things has not so much helped me to overcome this burden as it has served to increase my inner conflict with regard to reconciling my humanity.

I want so badly to be strict and disciplined enough to set balance to my world, if only in my near vicinity, but I am such a clichéd human myself that the cards seem always stacked against my breaking even with my environment. Left to my own devices, I might like to live in my own personally made Earthship as far from the hive as possible and coexist with my "yard" rather than trying to control it. However, I would do anything for my wife's continued acceptance and companionship, including living in the suburbs and making like I care what my neighbors think of my yard. The best compromise I can think to make is to be as conscientious a homeowner as possible with regard to things like pest control, sourcing of goods and building materials, and disposal of waste.

I want to reduce the number of felled trees my existence represents, but finding a natural alternative to toilet paper that is safe for modern plumbing and available throughout the seasons is too complicated to juggle with everything else and risks losing me the acceptance I crave from the humans around me;

not to mention I just so much love making things out of wood. The best I may do is to not be careless about my use of paper products and to source my wood materials from scrap, as much as possible. I utilize the material in my ever-evolving scrap wood pile at home to supplement my building projects, and when it gets whittled down to little bits, I trim them into door-stops and incorporate them into art pieces. My sons have grown into a love for welding, forging, and blacksmithing, leading us to practice similar cycling with our scrap metals.

I would also love to reduce my materialism, but I want to live a rich and fulfilled life, which entails trying out all the cool new toys and always wearing different clothes so the humans around me don't perceive me to be dirty. My compromise is to work my material goods until they have absolutely no functional value remaining whatsoever—from my clothing to my tools to my vehicles—and reuse, repurpose, and fix everything, whenever possible, rather than simply disposing of it because that's easier. At home I wear my clothing to tattered rags before literally repurposing them as rags and shop towels, leading me to constantly ride the fine line between *still useful* and *acceptable in appearance*, if only to my sweet wife.

I wish to be kind and accepting to the other life around me, but beyond the sustenance of my life requiring the death of other lives, I also instinctively crave to hunt. I do my best by consciously considering the heft of each life that must be extinguished in my daily bustling, by hunting responsibly and by choosing never to take a life senselessly. Much as I enjoy the thrill of any good hunt, for the sake of my biological conscience I prefer to hunt renewable things rather than extinguishing singular lives, which deprive other individuals of any of *their* time on Earth. One of my favorite things to hunt for are mushrooms and truffles—which are only small pieces of the organisms that produce them—but I can find a satisfying thrill in hunting many other things, from rocks and shells to mineral deposits or lost treasures, naturally shed elk antlers, medicinal plants (from which I harvest only pieces), and, of course, adventures.

I want to believe that our collective biological conscience will one day lead us all to choose, as a species, to cease the behaviors that are rapidly deteriorating the quality of life for all living things on planet Earth, but until that day, I, too, shamefully continue to operate and maintain multiple fossil-fueled internal combustion engines.

In society, I feel that we all share some degree of personal responsibility to prevent the spread of carelessness around ourselves, by giving those around us words of encouragement and praise for what they do well, especially when we bear witness to their times of struggle. Carelessness is the hindrance responsible for many individuals never even acknowledging their potential, much less achieving it. To live with purpose, we must learn to see carelessness and other detrimental attitudes for what they are and to break our own personal bonds to them.

Although it is *possible* to do this, no matter how much we like or dislike the tasks we find ourselves responsible for in any given moment of life, it is much easier to demonstrate care for what we are doing when we *want* to be doing it; giving it our actual best is pretty much impossible if we *do not want* to be doing it at all. For instance, if I should find myself participating in a relationship I do not want to be in but remain in anyway—for the sake of conflict avoidance, possible financial detriment, or whatever other excuse could be contrived—it can never grow into a better relationship, since I will always subconsciously hold back some degree of my care in every action. The same may be said for every job, family, friend circle, or any other social environment that I do not want to be in but choose to be in anyway. Instead, I choose to do things I *want* to be doing, so I may give them the care that will make them all that they may be—and in doing so, my life, in turn, becomes all that it may be. This goes hand in hand with maintaining my set of goals, both short and long term.

To me, goals are like a carrot, baited on a hook and made to hang just in front of a donkey's nose—from a pole mounted on its back—such that the donkey can't resist walking forward in an attempt to attain the carrot. We are like a donkey, in that our lives progress in a plodding fashion, one day after the next, for what seems an eternity. Finding goals to bait on our hooks that we find attractive enough to lead us on, day by day, is important so that one day we will look back at our lives without the regret of having done things we did not want to, or having done nothing at all.

When I am presented with an opportunity that looks particularly bright and shiny (that is, I would really *want* to do it), I put it on my hook and do what it takes to attain it. In this way, I may be led to an ever-shinier carrot as my life progresses. When I realize the carrot I have been trudging toward is rotten (I would *not want* to do it), I take it off my hook and find something better to bait myself with. I don't hesitate or procrastinate in this, for every moment I live in pursuit of this rotten carrot is another moment that my life could have been spent moving in the direction of a beautiful, glorious whopper of a carrot instead. If I do not want to be doing what I am doing, I stop doing it and go find something I want to do enough that I can bring myself to care about it, so I may be proud of my accomplishments and grow and maintain my self-respect.

I am fortunate that I have somehow always known I wanted to have children and also that my primary interest in this world is the life-forms inhabiting it. My whole life long, I have watched as most of the humans around me have struggled to attain even a wisp of the certainty I have about what it is they want to do with their given time to live. I have recently coached Zakai through this as he had just settled into an adult lifestyle and was uncertain in what direction his day-to-day life should proceed, and why.

Without being sure what he wanted to do and without the confidence of having done many things, he had been stuck in a sort of limbo, waking up early every day only to spend hours internalizing all of this uncertainty until it built up into a mental wall of hesitation that prevented him ever actually *doing* anything. Then he went to work for the night, got up the next day and started it all over again.

I pointed out to him what he was doing—because he was not aware of it—then explained that, for most people, discovering what they want to do requires that they first get out there and have some diverse experiences. In a world that is essentially infinite—from our perspective—choosing what we want to do

47

requires that we first familiarize ourselves with some sample set of possible activities from which we might choose or build on.

So long as he continued to spend his time not doing anything, Zakai was caught in a catch-22 in which he could not figure out what to do without knowing what his options might look like, but he could not know his options because he was not getting out there to discover them. I told him about a mantra I learned at Nick's Fishmarket on Maui in my youth: *anticipation, not hesitation.*

Nick's is a tightly run, fine-dining restaurant, operating on what is referred to in the industry as a captain system. All dining room staff begin at the bottom rung of a rank system and work their way up, competing with their peers to attain the next rung through study and practice of service techniques. Sections are 12 to 13 tables large, and teams consisting of rovers, bussers, back waiters, and front waiters coordinate service, with assistance from captains. The hot line in the kitchen—from which the food is organized systematically onto carts to be hustled out into the dining room—is a good 20 strides through a winding hallway packed crisply with service stations, and the nightly rigama-role happens at a breakneck pace. Everyone begins as a stocker, standing in the hallway polishing every last piece of silver and china as it flows incessantly from the kitchen dishwashing station.

Because the setup and service of food, cocktails, espresso, and everything else was so mechanistic, we were all trained to become faster and faster at each task but in a concise and efficient way, without becoming rushed or sloppy. Night by night, we all became extremely proficient at these tasks in our desire to outcompete one another for a chance at the next opening in the rank above.

The idea behind *anticipation, not hesitation* was that, while we were doing the task at hand just as quickly and proficiently as we could, in our minds we were anticipating what we would do next, so we never stopped to waste a moment hesitating. As it applied to my son's particular case, I reminded him that tomorrow morning would certainly find him beginning his same old mental routine upon waking, so he should anticipate it by planting for himself a trig-ger. I told him to imagine as vividly as he could that it *is* that moment tomorrow morning—which he knows will come—but imagine, when he begins to do the usual routine, catching himself and instead getting up out of bed right away to begin doing something else, thereby breaking the habit of lying there in hesitation. I asked him to anticipate now what he might want to do with the beginning of his day—before he went to work the following morning—and to add the first few steps of it to his vividly imagined trigger. I told him to imagine it one more time just before he fell asleep.

The next morning, when I awoke, he had already been on an adventure out in the world and returned to sink his teeth into a bunch of other things he had been procrastinating in the name of his chronic hesitations. Now he feels much more accomplished and better about himself and how he is spending his time.

Planting a mental trigger for myself is one technique I have learned that prevents me from becoming stagnant, but I first developed it to curb my own tendency to procrastinate. Procrastination is when I know I have something I should do but continue to put it off until later, for whatever reason. Habitual procrastination leads me to personal stagnation, in which I feel incapable of moving forward in my life because I have procrastinated so much. I convince myself that I am too busy or that other things are more important, but these excuses are the vehicles to my own self-enabling. I am the only one who may break this mental bad habit for myself. Learning how to avoid this for myself also began at Nick's, where complacency was the enemy. There I learned that procrastination, the first domino leading to complacency, occurs the very first time I become conscious of that thing I need to do and choose to walk past it instead of *doing something* about it.

At Nick's, because all of our tasks were fairly small, we were taught to do them as fast as we could think of them and not to walk past *anything* that needed doing. Of course, the rest of life is not restaurant work, so I have learned to adapt this idea to longer tasks by having the self-discipline to *do something* about that thing I might otherwise walk past. If it is a relatively large task, I either do a percentage of it before moving on or I act on it by putting it on a list I carry with me. If my lists are not with me, then I write initials representing it on the back of my hand, where I will see it often and transfer it to a list later or be spurred to get back to it in some other way, when I can.

I have further applied this technique to ideas that come to me in the course of my life, as doing nothing about them increases the probability they will not come to pass, while acting on them in some way allows me to pluck them from the unending stream of consciousness and coax them into being. I have found writing them on a calendar to be a useful tool for this.

I will do small tasks in their entirety when I come to be aware of their need to get done, but I also plant seeds for myself so I do not forget to take care of tasks that require action at an appropriate later time. For example, if I am busy doing something and Eleanor asks me to please drop packages at the post office for her later, when I go to work, I have learned that just acknowledging her verbally will certainly find me kicking myself later for having forgotten them and therefore not having been true to my word. Instead, I take the packages from her and place them on top of my work shoes or walk them out and place them on the driver's seat of my truck, so I may not get out the door without them. I have proven to be so easily distracted that even with these strategies, I still sometimes forget to make the stop and drop them off. I have further learned to place a package in my lap while I drive, or even on the dashboard in front of me, if I should happen to be particularly distractible on a given day. The more it is in my way now or in the way of my anticipated future self, the more likely I will not forget it.

Aside from learning coping strategies to avoid our own innate tendencies holding us back, to live with purpose we must also discover the purpose for which we find ourselves here, now. Although I have always known I wanted to have children and study life, it took me satisfying these desires for many years before I realized the larger purpose for which I believe I was born into this life at this particular time and place in history.

Having spent my formative years being mostly neglected by my human family and finding acceptance instead among the critters of the woods, I have always felt that the critters *were* family to me. As my life in human society has progressed, I have grown ever more ashamed of my human counterparts for their general lack of care, concern, and respect for the other critters of the planet and—in some ways even more—for one another.

In college biology classes, I learned that all of the other critters of the planet—be they flora, fauna, or fungus—*are our genetic relatives*, and I began to understand my personal feelings of deep kinship with them. Unfortunately, much as I had hoped that studying biology might find me surrounded by other like-minded, critter-loving hippies, my classmates—both students and instructors—found themselves there either for financial reasons or out of familial expectation. I was dismayed to witness a now-familiar human callousness toward the Earth's other organisms, even in my critter-centered classes.

I realized toward the end of my undergraduate studies that part of my purpose in this life is to confer some of my critter empathy to the humans around me. My hope in this is that, through a ripple effect, those to whom I am able to rub off an understanding of our deep ecological and ancestral connection to the other creatures of the world will one day contribute to a more holistically coexistive and sustainable human future than what I find myself living in today.

I spent four years developing and teaching a three-term biology basics class for children ages five to seven within my sons' homeschool community. A number of my students requested an advanced class, so Eleanor and I led a field research team of children eight to twelve years old in an independent research study of food preference among the crows of our neighborhood. We have since moved away and our kids have mostly grown up, but I still find many ways to instill in those around me the ideals I feel responsible to share; this book is one example.

Figuring out how best to nourish my soul has been a vital part of learning to live a life with purpose because I thrive on responsibilities and, as they say, to best take care of others, I must first take care of myself. My soul feels most content in the forest, so I choose to live near one and spend a lot of time there, especially in times of strife or frustration, when my way seems most unclear.

When Rachel passed, she left a book behind that eventually found its way into my hands, called *Be Here Now*, by Dr. Richard Alpert (now renamed Baba Ram Dass). It is a deeply spiritual book, depicting the author's journey of transformation from the lost, Western-educated doctor of medicine he had found himself to be, into the Eastern spiritual pupil he somehow knew he was always supposed to become—by way of a bottle of LSD and a walking journey through India. At the end of his experience, the single most important thing he needed to change about himself to become his most potent spiritual self was to learn to *be here now* all of the time, as deeply and sincerely as possible. This meant filtering out all the distractions of what had been, had not been, should have been, or would or would not come to be for the sake of giving his very best to every moment, as it was presented to him, with utmost presence of mind. This was how he learned to give his *time alive* the respect of sincere appreciation it deserved.

Being present-minded to my here and now has proven equally powerful for navigation of myself through this life, as the universe is constantly presenting opportunities for me to choose, both subtle and overt. If I am distracted, the probability that I will miss an important road sign of my life is much higher than if I am present-minded.

For this same reason, being happy, taking pride in doing my best, and feeling good about myself aids in maintaining the mental clarity required to keep my mind open to all of my options. On the other hand, being unhappy, being not proud for not doing my best, and feeling bad about myself contributes tremendously to the nagging mental distractions that result in unnoticed opportunities passing me by. For a more comprehensive look at reading and following your life's road signs, I recommend *The Celestine Prophecy*, a book by James Redfield.

Acutely focusing our attention on what we are doing in the present actually improves our body's visual, auditory, and olfactory acuity so that we are empowered to truly do our best while also being prevented from fretting neurotically over all of the many distractions that might otherwise detract from our performance. Probably the most common of these distractions is the tendency to stress over what uncertainties are yet to come or to worry over events that have already transpired. I try my best to be deliberate with my attention in every moment, so everything I do gets done as well as I may do it, for the sake of my own pride and self-respect but also to have the most concise effect possible on the world around me. As I see it, if I have decided something is worth doing at all, then to me it is worth doing as well as I am capable of doing it.

I have found that *being here now* is particularly important to woods navigation, wherein paying enough attention to tease subtle landmarks from the seemingly uniform environment is essential to keeping my bearings, deducing the most efficient path to my destination, and ensuring I get home in a timely manner. Bringing my critter and plant identification books into the wild with me on forays saw me arriving home late countless times, until I finally learned to bring the samples home instead. Disorientation in an unfamiliar place is all but certain after looking up from being absorbed in a book about the intricate technicalities of something else entirely.

A brief note on the topic of fear before I move on to the workout. Fear is an emotion induced by the perception of threat or danger, whether real or imagined. Like our stress responses, its physiological expressions are diverse and plentiful, but from my observations, the most common human response to fear in our modern world is a lack of action. When considering an attempt at a task perceived to be difficult, the fear of failing—in any of a plethora of conceivable ways—makes it easier to decide against attempting at all, and even more so the more time we spend reconsidering it, as we may just continue conceiving of them.

For many of us, it need not only be a fear of failure that prevents us from acting but could be simply the fear of *not knowing* what the outcome will be of our conjectured desire. Fear of the dark is the most basic example of this, as the dark may hold a vast wonderland of glorious treasures just as well as it might contain some nasty monster, but for some reason, our human minds tend toward the presumption of the latter. Perhaps it is because it makes choosing inaction so much easier rather than risking anything at all in going to find out.

Learning to confront and overcome my fears one at a time throughout my life as I become aware of them allows me to drive out personal insecurities and to become more confident about handling future unknowns. I have found success in overcoming my own fears through a conscious recognition that the more fear I allow myself, the less rich my life becomes and that, in this life, nothing good comes easy.

What I mean is, when I take on something I think of as difficult and succeed in doing it, I tend to value the experience and whatever came of it much more than if it were just given to me. Having to try hard to attain something seems automatically to confer a greater intrinsic value to it, while experiences and opportunities I am just given—or told I have to do, making them obligatory— tend to be more easily taken for granted or treated carelessly. This applies to both things I was born into and things that have been given to me, in the hands I am dealt on the daily.

My experiences with confronting and overcoming my own fears have taught me that the worst that may come of my blazing confidently into the dark to illuminate the unknown is that I may make some mistakes. Since mistakes represent the experience I gained when I didn't get what I wanted, what I learn from them advances my life more than if I had instead allowed fear to prevent me from acting at all. Additionally, whatever shakes out of the experience will seem more valuable to me for having made the effort, and it tends to lead my mind to consider what to do next as a result of this new experience and the confidence gained from it.

My life's experiences have taught me that we have no guarantees. We may spend our entire lives living with the recklessness of a death wish only to die of ripe old age, or we may live our whole lives in utter reserve, holding back in hopes of avoiding negative consequences, only to have our lives spontaneously and unpredictably cut short by unforeseen circumstances. I have learned from these observations that spending my life dwelling on what the universe is going to do in response to my actions is senseless and only leads me to the frustration of disappointed expectations. I seek to live without fear or expectation, considering the occurrences of my life with an open heart and learning from them what I may, while simply doing my best in every moment. Living my life in fear, for any period of time, reduces the potential for it to be brilliant and amazing, so I have made a personal pact with myself to confront and drive out any fears I may have the very moment I become aware of them.

I believe this is the only opportunity I will ever have to live, which means that for me, every opportunity I am presented with is also the *only* chance I will ever get to have that particular experience, in just that way. I choose to live my life *like I mean it*, without carelessness, fear, or *I can'ts* because it might well be my only one. I remain ever-conscious of the fact that everything may always become worse than it is for me right now to make the best of every hand I am dealt so as not to find myself looking back, in my moment of death, at a life lived in regret.

In the words of my old kiteboarding guru, Stan, "If I die with even an ounce left to give, I will not have lived life full enough!"

SECTION 2: THE WORKOUT

I learned about our body's energy budget in college biology. The basic idea is that for organisms to persist, they must consume more calories from their food than they expend to acquire and process it. Our human bodies were evolved to travel miles and miles by foot each day, hunting and gathering food gradually along the way. However, in this modern world, virtually no output of calories is required to rustle up a meal of any size. This has led us to a population-wide lack of caloric common sense, propagating our nation's growing obesity epidemic and making many other conditions of physiological imbalance downright commonplace.

A regular workout is an acknowledgment that our modern human bodies exist far outside of the context for which, and in which, they were custom-evolved to fit. Keeping a naturally balanced calorie and activity budget involves a set of instinctive behaviors that we as modern humans must reawaken and choose to maintain for our human organism to be healthy.

I have developed my personal workout routine with the conscious intention of regularly engaging and strengthening every muscle group in my body while sustaining a high degree of flexibility and metabolic flow through them. My goal is to stave off the muscular complacency that might eventually limit my daily activities—by way of cramping or general weakness—as well as to achieve and retain the greatest strength and in the greatest range of motion possible, throughout my body. In this way, I diminish the probability that any of life's challenges might prevent my natural progression, so I may be empowered to do my very best at whatever I desire to accomplish.

Although my habit now is to work out every other day, when I was young I did it much more often because my body told me it needed it. I would often find myself jumping up at two o'clock in the morning—from a so-far sleepless rest—to pump out some intensity (sometimes for the third time in a day) so my body could be tired enough to finally let my mind drift off to sleep. Whatever the frequency, the most important thing has always been for me to listen to my body.

Because I have developed my routine outside the constructs of social constraints, I did not know the names attributed to many of my workout motions until researching to write this book, and for some, I have been unable to find labels previously applied to them. For the sake of you, my human audience, I have attempted to incorporate the terms used by other humans previously in describing particular motions as I go through them.

CHAPTER 3
Finding the Motivation

In my observation of others, it strikes me that finding motivation is the biggest hindrance to both beginning a workout routine and continuing to keep up with it.

At around ten years old, I began to experience chronic debilitating back and neck outages, to the extent that I missed school regularly for not being able to turn my head from the side I woke up with it on. My father took me to a string of naturopathic specialists who had varying success working out the issue at hand, much less any leads on what was causing it or how to prevent it from happening again. Finally, just before my 13th birthday, he took me to a wise old osteopath who ordered a full set of back and neck X-rays before explaining that I had been born with a couple of skeletal defects, namely moderate scoliosis and two fused and offset vertebrae in my neck.

"Young man," he told me, "from this day forward, you have a choice: you may do nothing different and be forever plagued by these issues of symmetry, or you may adopt a regular, symmetrical workout routine—so that your muscles may keep your bones straight—and you might one day have the chance to lead a normal life." He sent me home with a basic beginning calisthenics instruction pamphlet and a handful of one-inch rubber lifts to wear in my left shoe. I promptly lost the lifts, as I was a hippie-raised young boy who went barefoot exclusively or wore flip-flops, at most, when I had to for school, but I did take the workout advice to heart and began building my routine in earnest.

This has always been my biggest motivator, as all it takes is a week or so without working out for my body to be wracked with kinks and cricks again. I think of it as staving off the crooked, hunchback body I feel creeping in on me if I do not keep up with it. Although not everyone has a built-in negative reinforcer like me, we do each have our own personal physical challenges to overcome, every one of which represents an opportunity for motivation, since physical debilitations tend to worsen with atrophy and improve with strengthening.

Over the years, I have learned many other good reasons to maintain a regular workout regime. It gives me the ability to channel daily stress into productivity instead of letting it build into periodic outbursts. For me, the days that have the most stress—or even just the most stressful single events in them—are the days my workouts are strongest, and if I am unable to make time for it on such a day, I will consciously subdue my stress response to channel it into my next workout.

It also functions as an immediate immunity boost by increasing overall physiological function via increased circulation, respiration, and metabolic flow. When I begin to perceive my body coming down with an illness or I am just not feeling strong for my day's planned activities, I knock out a quick, intense workout to give me whatever edge I need. Also, continuing to work out through sickness—even increasing the frequency, if I feel able—means I kick it sooner and come out of it stronger than I was to begin with.

If there's no good reason why I should not work out on a given day, I make sure to do it because there's no telling the future, and tomorrow something may come that actually prevents me from getting to it. In this way, I blaze through my life, having an illness that actually stops my productivity only once every few years.

Working out is also a direct tool for building self-confidence, as my choice to prove to myself that I *can* complete each individual muscle contraction (termed rep, short for repetition) in every sequential set (series of reps) builds my belief in myself that I *can* do what I believe I can. When confronted with a particularly daunting physical task, I often do a preliminary, confidence-building workout first, to increase the probability I will absolutely knock it out of the park.

In every life, some pain will inevitably come, if only through growth and development. We each must choose whether we allow that pain to hold us back or leverage it to drive us forward. What does not kill me truly does make me stronger, not only in the physical sense—with my muscles literally tearing and scarring to grow bigger—but also mentally and emotionally. This means that allowing some pain to prevent me from *doing* sets me up for a diminishing sense of "I can" in addition to the muscular atrophy my body experiences from actually doing less. A life that seeks to avoid all pain and discomfort is destined for some disappointment, so I choose to set myself up for success by deciding it is a driving force in my life. I feel most capable when I am pushing hard enough in every workout to maintain a small degree of muscle soreness all over, every day.

I remember my aunt Jeanette visiting when I was 13 or so and a conversation we had just after she watched me run a crazy, high-energy street basketball game. She's a nurse and said that in her experience with people and life, when it comes to your energy, if you don't use it, you will eventually lose it. I learned from this to be an aggressive doer of all of the many things I am driven to do in my life and not to relax this attitude as age naturally slows my pace. I have watched the natural energy levels of those around me decline with disuse as life has passed, while I have continued to run ever-faster circles around my own kids, even as they have grown into adults. I attribute this primarily to my regular workouts maintaining a high metabolic momentum in my body; that is, because I make sure to still use my energy, I still have it *to use*.

In Oregon, where I live, winters are fairly cold, so I do a lot of what I call *workout for warmth* through the fall and winter, to maintain a high immune response and stave off the planet's seasonal attempts to put a lid on my energy level. People who are chronically cold or suffer from seasonal depression would benefit from a regular morning routine through the dismal days of fall and winter, both physically and spiritually. I tend to work out harder and more often during the winter months to keep the juices flowing, and skip more sessions in the summer months, when more active real-life opportunities abound.

I have always been someone who thrives on responsibilities and love showing how much responsibility I may handle for those I care about. I was especially this way when our kids were little and all of life seemed to be an intense test of mental endurance. As a result, there have been a couple of times when I have come to feel overwhelmed with the sense that I have no time left for me to do anything *for myself.* Carving out my 30 minutes to work out at least every other day has served to stave off that feeling indefinitely, as it is something I do *exclusively for me.*

All of these are good motivators for maintaining the strongest body I can and also culminate in a bigger-picture motivation as well. With all of the *I can'ts* pushed out and the most potent physical self possible being maintained as a normal condition, nothing stops me from taking whatever opportunities come my way in daily life, leading to a more fulfilling existence that continues to build in vigor.

My workout empowers my life's activities, and my activities, in turn, hone the efforts of my workout. I am careful not to get into the habit of thinking that because I am working out so strongly and regularly, other physical activities are, therefore, unnecessary. It takes both to evince my brightest life.

CHAPTER 4
Mechanics: The When and How

Before the old doctor, all I knew about working out came from the traditional posturing and hazing of junior high gym class, and so I followed his pamphlet, strictly. At the time, I was a poor, scrawny white boy with glasses who just wanted to play basketball and certainly needed some muscles to drive my desires.

By the time I discovered the weight room in high school gym class, I had long since hit the ceiling with my pamphlet exercises and gone ahead and ramped them up with lots of extra sets of push-ups and sit-ups. Eager for more, I became a real regular in the weight room, pushing out all that strong young man energy and truly surging with the vigor of youth.

I remember—during my senior year—having one of those stereotypical football coaches of a health instructor, Mr. Patterson, who said something on the first day of his class that has stuck with me ever since. He shared with us a statistic he said he would like for us to avoid: that the average American is in the best shape of their lives during their senior year of high school. This bit of information motivated me to be in the best shape of my life every sequential year from then until the reduced elasticity of age checked me hard at age 30.

There have been a few times in my life when I have had to stop working out, like when I got my hernia and when I was bedridden for weeks figuring out my stress disorder. Starting back up again took a bit of preliminary consideration because my routine had been gradually built up over the course of my adult existence and did not begin from such a zero point. However, I feel this experience—of beginning from a point of severe atrophy and complete loss of habit—is a good blueprint for beginning to develop one's own workout habits from scratch. So, for the sake of those whom it may benefit, I describe the motions of each muscle group from this perspective as I go over my routine.

Although I have never officially received one, my high-energy impulsiveness and difficulty focusing through my thoughts on the here and now would make me a prime candidate for an ADHD diagnosis, like so many of us in this hyperactively overstimulating modern world. Expecting myself to remember—as the days of my life pass by—whether I did upper body in my last workout or lower body, or biceps versus triceps, or whatever, has only ever served to confuse me. For this reason, I simply work out my entire body in every workout.

Core

The core of our bodies consists of everything in the midsection, including the front, sides, and back. Not only is our core the intersection of all of our body parts, joining together everything else, it is also tied into so much of the rest of our musculature that most sizable movements incorporate some degree of core. For this reason, I consider in this section exercises focusing primarily on the midsection, although I am aware that many others engage the core as well.

In the beginning, when core strength is weak, I find a good starting point is simply to lie flat on my back with my knees up, as in a sit-up position. I do as many reps as I feel able to, just flexing my abdominals and holding for a moment, focusing on pressing my lower back to the floor as I flex.

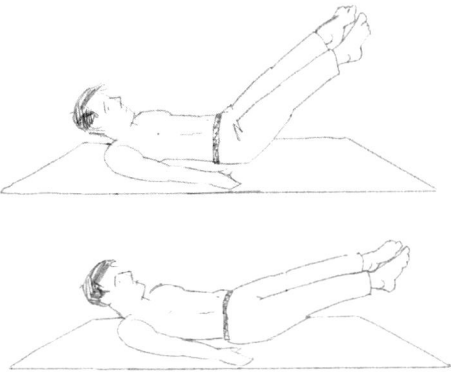

[figure1]

I alternate these with sets of as many simple leg lifts (figure 1) as I can muster, and I increase their range of motion and number as I get stronger. If I am not able to lift my legs yet, I will flex my abdominals with legs held rigidly straight, gradually increasing reps and hold time, until I am able to lift them, even just a tiny bit, then I build on that.

I feel that no simulated workout motion could ever compete with any real-world work affecting the same muscle group, so while I am doing my sets, I often imagine that I am doing some real-world activity that engages the same area.

For leg lifts, I think back to my time playing soccer, when we would all take turns standing over one another and pushing each others' legs back down as they came up, for the sake of added resistance. As we each got stronger, we would begin to alternate from lifting our legs straight up to lifting them back and forth, from one side to the other (figure 2), to increase range of motion and tie more core strength into other muscle groups.

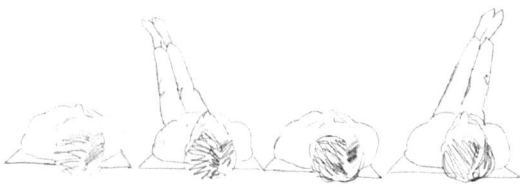

[figure2]

After a few workouts, when these motions begin to feel easy, I change just flexing abdominals into doing crunches (figure 3). I discovered quickly that doing crunches with my hands cradling my head—as I had seen other people do—caused me to experience chronic neck sprain, so I have always preferred to do them with my hands out in front of me instead. I think of my hands as a counter-weight, subtly increasing or decreasing resistance, depending on whether I am holding them to my chest, as far as I can ahead of myself, or anywhere in between. I use the positioning of my hands to increase resistance as I build up strength over time.

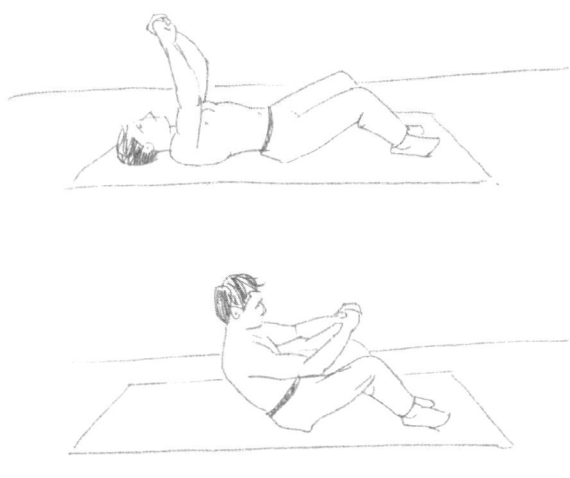

[figure3]

I am conscious not to fling my hands out ahead of myself, as the momentum used to complete the motion increases the probability that I may hurt my neck. It also detracts from the development of my abdominals, of course. I find it is much better to go slow and steady in the beginning, learning to do each motion properly, until I get stronger and may then increase my pace without using momentum.

As far as numbers go, I begin wherever I feel comfortable and just keep adding more and more as time goes by and my muscles get stronger. If a day comes in which I do not feel strong enough to hit the numbers I had expected to, I do not beat myself up because I know other days will come, and doing what I *am* able to do is far better than doing nothing at all. By the same token, if one day I reach my target number and feel like I could just keep on going, then I do, because my body is clearly ready to advance.

Unfortunately, as these middle years of my life have passed, the reduced elasticity of my body has forced a gradual decline in numbers and range of motion. Again, I am careful not to beat myself up about it, since it is only the natural process of time degrading my mechanistic body, and a refusal to acknowledge it will result in chronic injuries.

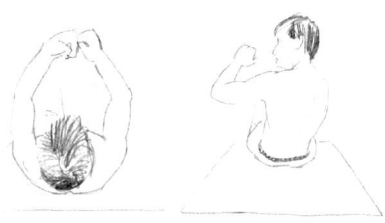

[figure4]

When some time has passed and crunches seem easy, I add in a set of side-to-side crunches (figure 4), and when they get boring, I add in some bicycle crunches (figure 5). While doing bicycle crunches, I like to think of the most intense uphill moments of a weeklong bike-packing trek I took with Dane for my 28th birthday. For the sake of my neck, I do not cradle my head in my hands while doing bicycle crunches, either.

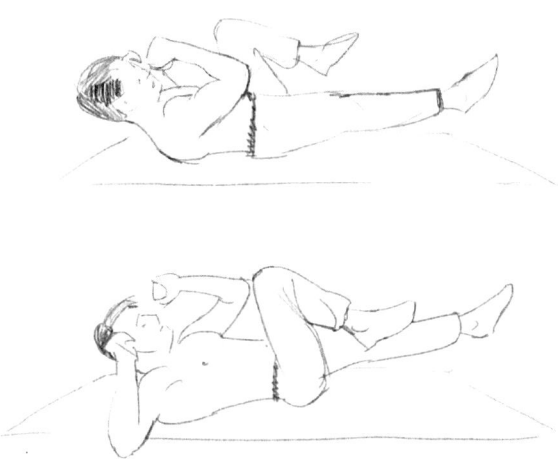

[figure5]

For the core area of my back, I lie on my stomach and do the Superman exercise (figure 6), raising my arms off the floor, out in front of me, while also raising my feet at the same time. In the beginning, when I am not so strong,

I just lie down in this position and alternate flexing and relaxing my erector spinae (back muscles, just along the sides of the spine) (figure 7). After a few workouts, I am able to lift my legs off the floor, and then—after more strengthening—my arms as well.

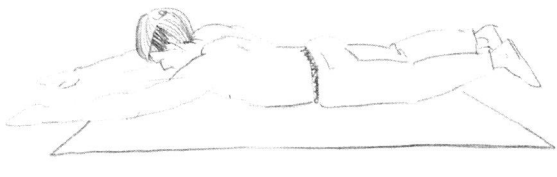

[figure6]

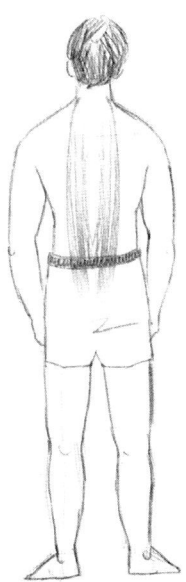

[figure7]

While doing this activity, I think of my time in college yoga class, where I learned to stretch my whole body into it—from tips of fingers to tips of toes—to maximize range of motion and build muscles that are long and lean, rather than short and stout. I believe this is better because longer, leaner muscles are more flexible and recharge faster than shorter, stouter ones, leading me to have fewer limitations in my daily life.

I focus on my hands and feet not touching each other since, when they do, they act as one unit, allowing the side of my body that is slightly stronger than the other to pull more weight, thereby keeping me strong in a lopsided way. Much of my routine is focused on this equilateral muscle-building so as to avoid subconsciously exacerbating my innately crooked frame. After a time, I begin to lift and hold for a count that gets progressively longer, and when I've built up enough strength to feel ready for advanced movements, I lift and lower in reps, just like crunches.

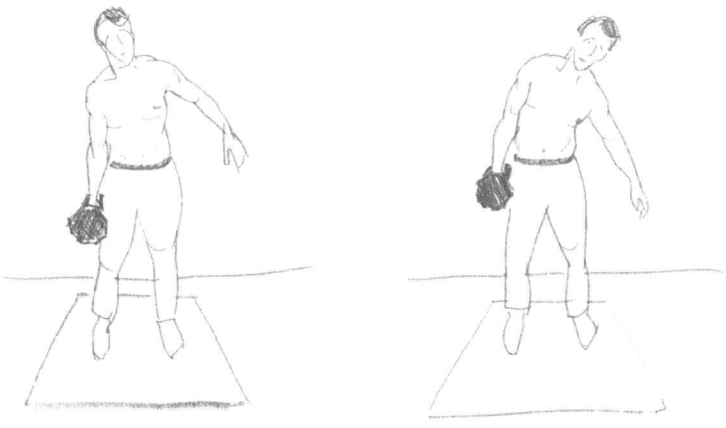

[figure8]

I do side bends for sides (figure 8) in my core area, which may be built up over time. I begin by standing up straight with my feet shoulder-width apart and drawing one hand down toward the floor—effecting a bend at my obliques (figure 9)—before slowly straightening back up to just past the starting position. After doing as many reps as I feel comfortable with, I switch and do the other side.

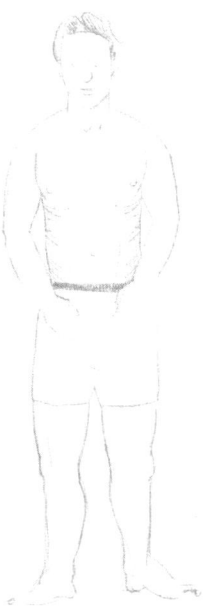

[figure9]

While doing this exercise, I think of carrying a five-gallon bucket full of water with one arm, to avoid my hand wandering too far out to the side because this creates a counter-weight effect that allows my body to cheat by relying on the support of surrounding muscle groups. I want to be as intently focused as possible on the muscle group I intend to be doing the work, isolating it to ensure I am truly making my body do what I want it to. This technical control of the body frequently comes in handy in my daily life, when I attempt something new or adapt to a change in the physical demands of achieving my goals, even in improving performance with activities I already do proficiently.

In the beginning, some compensation from other muscle groups is expected until I have built up the strength to be more focused on single muscles driving the motion. For this reason, it may feel as though I am just going through the motions for several sessions, until my muscles are developed enough that I may be consciously in touch with each one, individually.

When I have done enough side bends that they feel easy, I grab a lightweight dumbbell in one hand and let it pull that hand down to initiate the bend and give resistance against which to straighten back up. After as many of them as I can accomplish, I switch the weight to the other hand and do the same number of reps on the other side. Over time, I am able to gradually build strength by increasing the size of the weight I am holding, range of motion, and number of reps I do. With this exercise, I try to keep in the forefront of my mind that the muscle group I am working is actually the opposite side than that of the one holding the weight. I am essentially doing a side crunch, using the side opposite of the one that is weighted, to pull the weight back up.

Once my muscles are strong enough that I may focus conscious attention on the group I am working, I isolate them from the support of surrounding groups. Mirrors are an excellent tool for this because I am able to look directly at the muscles being worked, helping to intensify that conscious focus without having to crane my neck in ways that may lead to injury. If I am working a muscle or group I may not easily see—like my trapezius (figure 10), running down the sides of the spine from upper to mid-back—then I use my mind's eye to vividly imagine I am seeing that part of my body through the eyes of an observer.

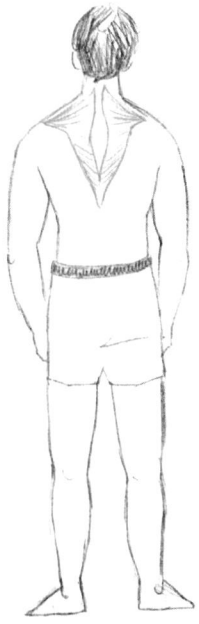

[Figure10]

I only added side bends in my late 20s, after a particular day in my job as a plywood plant worker. On this day, the foreman commissioned me with the task of driving the forklift, with a giant rubber floor-scraper attachment, to gather all the splinters from the floors all over the plant and feed them in bits to a ditch-like conveyor belt that carried them off to the paper mill. Where the conveyor belt left our building, the wall created a bottleneck, and I would have to get out of the forklift and take a long steel pole with a hook on the end to unjam stacks of splintered wood against constant upstream pressure from the unceasing belt. I unknowingly isolated my obliques as I pulled, pushed, and fussed with it, all day long. The next day, I was extremely sore in just my obliques, and it occurred to me that my workout routine needed amendment.

My workout is like an integrative reflection of the rest of my life, such that it empowers my life's activities while my activities, in turn, reinforce the efforts of my workout.

Lower Body

Lower body is everything below the waist—buttocks, thighs, calves, and feet—and as the driver of our primary means of locomotion, it is generally the region of our bodies that gets the most natural exercise, out of mere daily necessity.

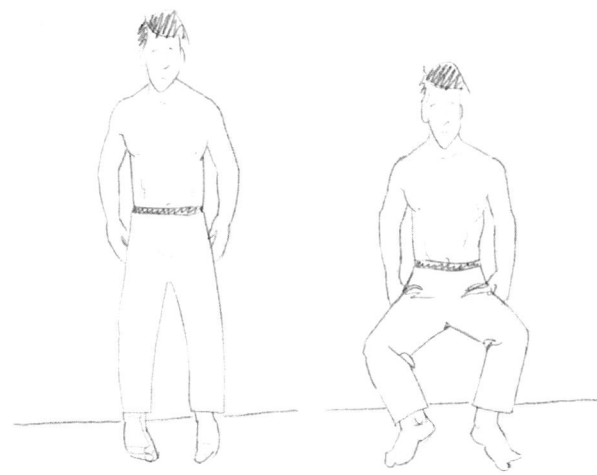

[Figure11]

73

When beginning to work this region, I first do wall-sits (figure 11), standing with my back against a wall, my feet shoulder-width apart, and heels about six inches away from the wall (or whatever is most comfortable). I bend slowly at the knees, allowing my upper body to slide down along the wall, as far as I feel able to, and hold for a count that leaves me with the energy to push myself back up again.

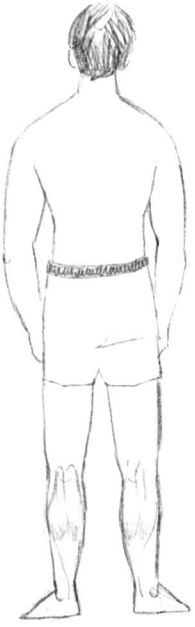

[Figure12]

I increase my count, one workout after another, until it gets boring, then I stop holding and instead slide down and pop back up, making it into reps that increase in range of motion and number with each session. I try to think of my body as a spring while I do this, taking on a load and slowly contracting as I slide down before springing back up again, like the load has been relieved. Also, to incorporate the calves (figure 12) and feet, I end in a calf raise (figure 13), so I finish my pop up on my toes and hold there for a moment before dropping back down for the next rep.

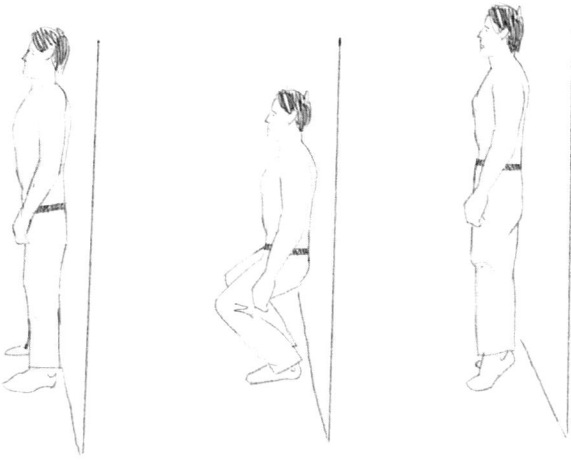

[figure13]

When the day comes that it seems too easy, I come away from the wall and do it, turning them into squats (figure 14). While doing squats, I focus on keeping my head up and my back straight, like a puppet with a string running straight through the center of the head all the way to the tailbone. When the day comes that this too gets tedious, I add equal-sized dumbbells in each hand, increasing their weight over time, as my strength grows.

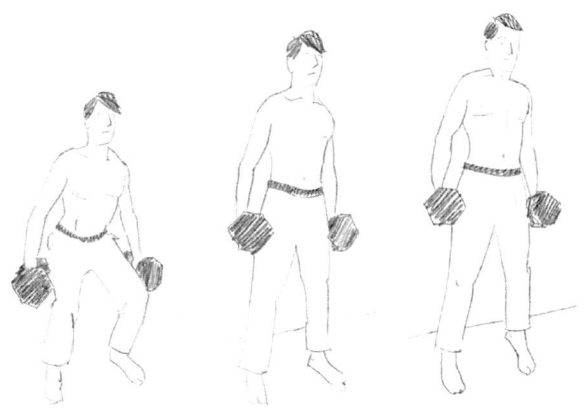

[Figure14]

Doing squats always reminds me of the two guys I used to see on the neighborhood basketball court who dreamed of being able to dunk off a feet-together jump from right under the hoop. I watched them—both on the court and in the weight room—as they made this dream come true, over the course of a year. Every day they were in the weight room, doing just what I have described above but with the addition of actually jumping off the ground with every pop. They spent all their time at the court practicing the same feet-together jump, from just under the hoop, getting steadily higher as their weights increased in the weight room, until they could both do it at will. Neither of them was even six feet tall, and these were your standard ten-foot-high rims. As someone who only ever cared to try and dunk the easy way—from a long, sailing, one-footed jump at high speed—it was remarkable to witness.

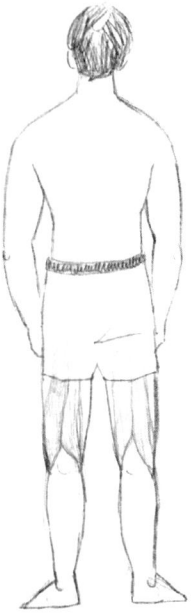

[figure15]

I continue to feel as though my hamstrings (figure 15) are not engaged by this activity as directly as the other muscles of my lower body, leading me to be aggressive about supplementing with real-life activities. Being hyperactive and living on a steep hillside—on which I personally carved our house out of years of neglected vegetation and am perpetually maintaining it amidst nearly an acre of ever-encroaching plant life—serves as a regular, real-life lower-body workout. Beyond that, my preferred supplemental real-life activities for engaging these muscles include snowboarding, skateboarding, surfing, kiteboarding, bicycling, and aggressive mountain climbing—but not the kind with ropes and rocks, rather the steep hiking kind. I am sure other humans with a different perspective from my own could conceive of many more.

Upper Body

Upper body consists of everything I have not already covered: arms, chest, shoulders, and upper back.

I do push-ups (figure 16) as an upper body warm-up because they activate all muscle groups without exhausting any of them, as weight cannot easily be added, only more reps completed. I start with easy ones, from my knees, when I am still building up strength, then graduate from my knees to my toes as time goes by and I get stronger. If I am weak when getting started, I may even have a couple workouts doing a simpler push-up-and-hold until I am able to do some reps.

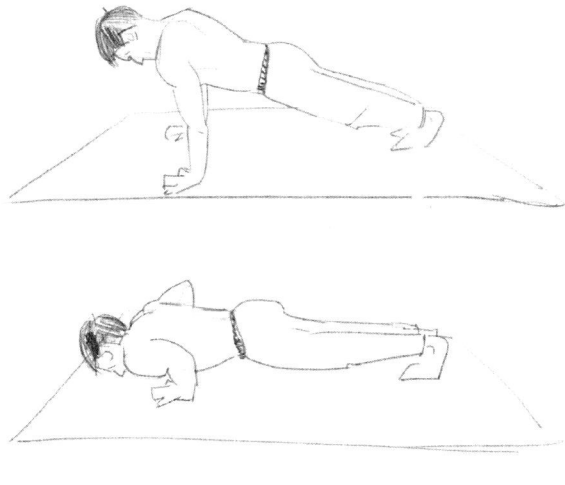

[figure16]

77

I slowly increase my range of motion as time passes until I am able to go down to the extent that my chest almost touches the floor. Eventually I vary them from one session to the next, alternating between hands at standard shoulder-width apart, to wide stance, to doing them on my knuckles (making my hands into fists). When I was young and played a lot of basketball, I would also include a small set on my fingertips, to strengthen the crispness of my shot.

Although I used to think of push-ups as upside-down bench presses—imagining I was pushing up a heavy bar full of weights—in recent years I have adapted a different visualization technique. I once heard a series of jokes about Chuck Norris, the legendary martial artist, all based on his well-known physical intensity. One joke, in particular, about how he does push-ups—pushing the Earth down rather than simply lifting himself up—has always stuck in my head. Now, I prefer to embody Chuck Norris while doing push-ups, thinking of my body as a fixed object in space and pushing the Earth away, rather than simply lifting my body up, which allows me to impart a greater degree of intensity to this exercise.

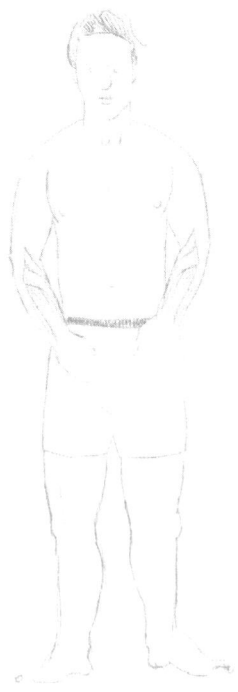

[figure17]

I do forearms (figure 17) next because I like to build in magnitude as I proceed through my workout, beginning with small muscle groups and moving into bigger ones as I get warmed up. Forearm muscles are divided into two groups: the ones on the underside for flexing the wrist and fingers inward, and the ones on the topside for extending them back out again.

Having always been naturally crooked, I have learned to ensure even development, as much as is possible, by allowing my weakest side to set the pace. No matter what, my stronger side will always be able to do the reps my weaker side can—in any given muscle group—but if I were to work my strong side first, I'd unnecessarily run the risk of doing more reps than my weak side may match, leading me to further unevenness. I extend this idea to everything I may think to, including forearms, by starting with the weaker topside so as not to burn my energy out on the naturally stronger, meaty underside first.

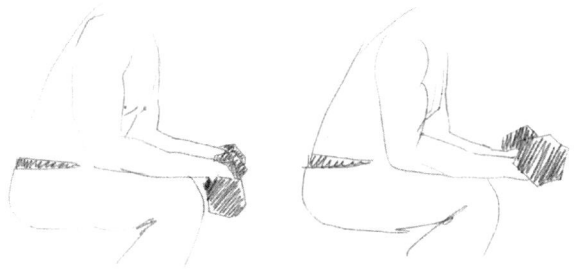

[figure18]

To begin, I sit on an unyielding chair or bench, rather than a cushy couch or bed, which allows my knees to make as close to a 90 degree angle as possible. Keeping my back straight, I bend forward at the waist until my forearms rest on top of my thighs and my hands and wrists hang out past my knees. I then rotate my forearms so my palms are facing the floor, and I allow my wrists to relax, hands hanging down. I then lift them up—from the wrist for their full range of motion—and hold them at the top before allowing them to slowly lower back down to their initial hanging position (figure 18). I am conscious to engage the posterior forearm muscles throughout the entire motion, but especially intensely during the hold-at-the-top phase. After doing as many reps of these as I feel capable of, I rotate my forearms so my palms are now up and repeat the motion as many times as I can (figure 19). To aid in maintaining symmetry, I imagine I am holding a long, straight bar with both hands—at about shoulder width from one another—which leads into adding dumbbells in both hands as time passes and I become strong enough to do so.

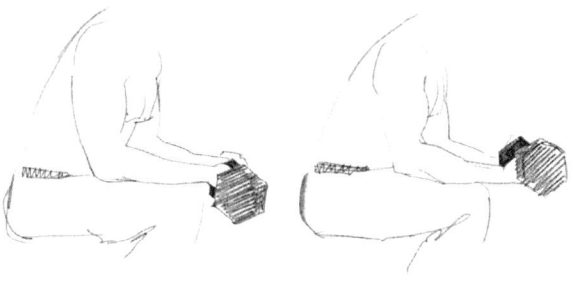

[figure19]

I like to think of forearms and other small muscle groups as being like "ones" in Yahtzee, in that they have only a small capacity to grow no matter how hard I may work them because they are innately smaller muscles to begin with. That said, my aunt Crystal, who has spent much of her life as a self-proclaimed career "washerwoman," has remarkably large and well-defined forearms—one of which is much larger on the topside, and the other on the underside—from years of wringing out towels and sheets in the same way, over and over again.

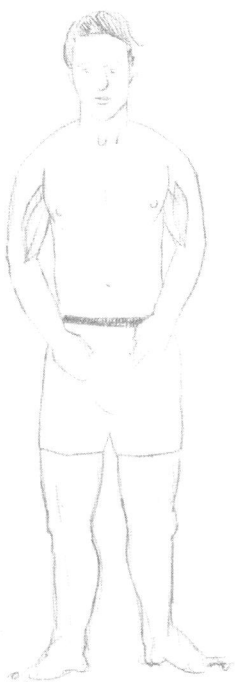

[figure20]

I also once knew a logger who had an otherwise inauspicious body but with downright comically large biceps (figure 20), and even more pronounced forearms, from years of holding down a large chainsaw, day after day. His markedly slight wrists will always serve as a reminder to me that our wrists—like our ankles, knees, and hips—are joints and therefore not able to be built up larger than they already are, as muscles may be. They must instead be strengthened by the building up of surrounding musculature, just like my crooked spine.

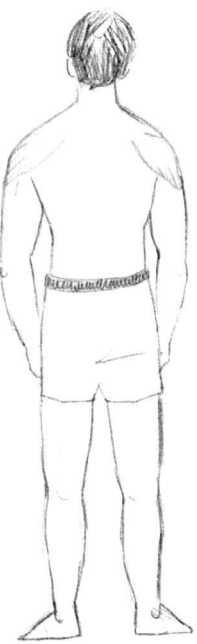

[figure21]

After forearms, I move into shoulders (figure 21), which in normal daily activity do much more supporting and tying together of other groups than being directly engaged, so I find myself inclined to spend more time on them in my routine. Because my shoulders have been separated so many times, I do more exercises with them now than I ever have in the past, to keep them strong for future injury prevention.

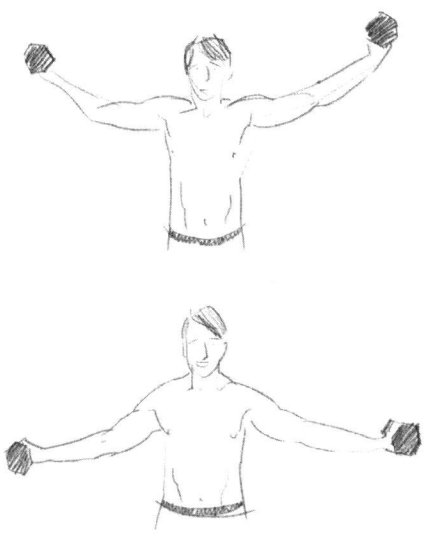

[figure22]

First, I stand up straight, with my head up and shoulders back, allowing my hands to hang at my sides. I lift both of my arms out to the sides at the same time (figure 22), in the fashion of a bird flapping its wings, which is what I vividly imagine I am while doing this activity. Bringing both arms up until they, together, create a line parallel to the horizon, with hands both at shoulder height, I begin my reps. I allow my hands to slowly drop, by about six inches, before raising them back up to about six inches above my horizon line. With time and strengthening, my range of motion increases, although never more than about a foot in either direction of the horizon line. Eventually, I add dumbbells.

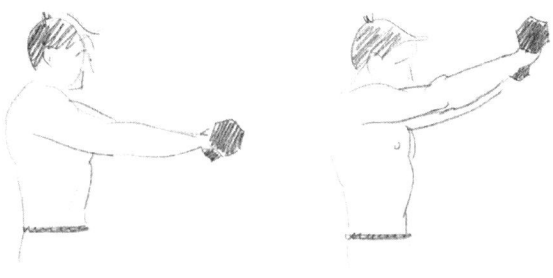

[figure23]

Next, I do anterior shoulder-raises (figure 23)—with my hands making their horizon line stretched out in front of me instead—being certain to keep my arms shoulder-width apart throughout the motion.

Then, I go into a simple, whole-shoulder movement that, in the upper body, looks just like I am swimming a front crawl stroke (aka Australian crawl). I remember doing a similar movement in yoga class, in which we held our arms out to the sides and traced first little circles with our hands and then big ones. We did sets in both a forward direction and then a backward direction, but this exercise is like big circles in the forward direction, with an initial draw backward that turns them into the emulation of a swimming stroke (figure 24).

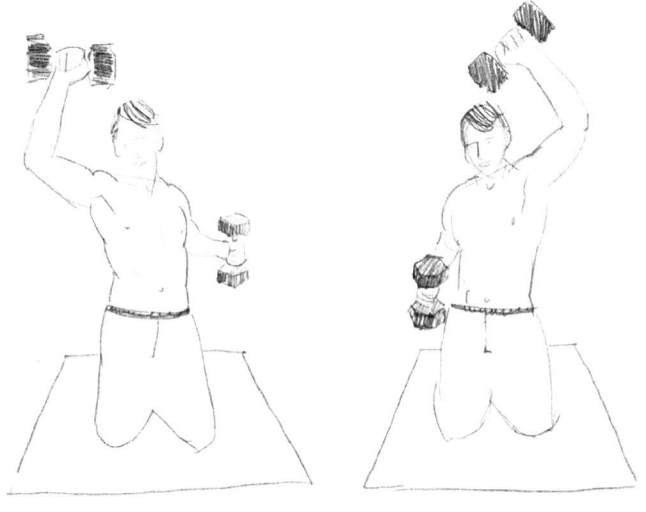

[figure24]

When I have a low ceiling to contend with, I will do all of these shoulder movements from my knees, with knees at least shoulder-width apart and back straight. After a time, I add equal dumbbells in each hand, but I remember, when initially adding and then increasing weight, to focus on not moving so fast that I allow my momentum to get me rocking, whether from side to side or from front to back.

As a young man living in Hawaii, I surfed as often as possible, and my workout consisted almost entirely of multiple variations of crunches and push-ups. Being a landlocked Idahoan by birth, I had never learned to swim and survived the Hawaiian surf by always wearing a surfboard leash and scrambling awkwardly back to my board every time I fell off. This all served me well enough until I moved to Florida, where the surf was absolutely miserable by comparison. Over the course of my first six months there, my lower back became ever weaker and more prone to chronic outages as my surf sessions dwindled.

The longer I lived in Florida, the more my lower back was chronically out because it became progressively weaker as my abdominals, on the *opposing* side of my trunk, were still being regularly strengthened. My brilliant wife pointed out that it was time for me to learn to swim, so I paid $20 for a one-hour personal swim lesson at my local YMCA. I spent the rest of my time in Florida with no lower back issues, catching weekly swim sessions at the plethora of public pools littered all around. My later move to Oregon prompted the addition of the Superman exercise for lower-back maintenance, as surf is even more miserable here and public pools are far fewer and farther between.

While doing my laps in the pool, submerging my face in the water provokes a strong fight-or-flight response from my body, which I then channel into intensity, imagining my biggest wave-riding sessions back in Hawaii. I tear up the pool so intensely that my first lap usually sees the exit of those in my neighboring lanes.

Now, as I push out my swim-like shoulder exercises against the resistance of 25-pound dumbbells in each hand, I imagine that I am swimming half of the mile-wide Columbia River, back to the safety of my home shore, against the pull of a barn-door-sized kite—bagging water like a fishing net—and my 14mm thick wetsuit, swollen with its own water weight. This being a circumstance I find myself in often, imagining it makes these exercises seem easy.

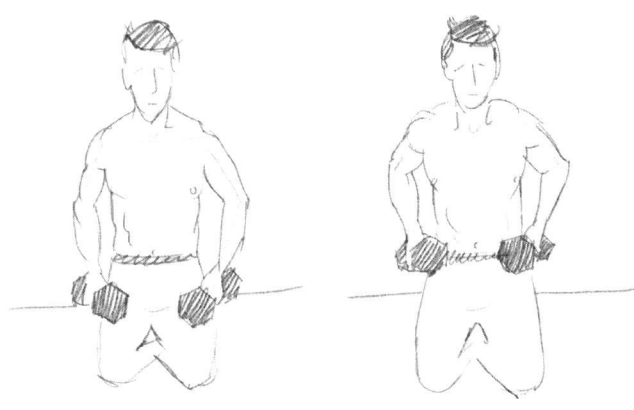

[figure25]

Shrugs (figure 25) are next, and they are just as simple as they sound. I begin by standing (or from my knees) with arms at my sides, head up and shoulders back, then shrug my shoulders as many times as I feel able to. This is another action that, at first, leaves me feeling like I am just going through the motions, but after a time I find my trapezius muscles become tight enough that I feel them flex as I go. When I get to this point, I begin to flex and hold them before relaxing them again. Then one day, after this has become easy, I add equal weights in each hand and continue. When graduating up to holding weights, no matter how small, I expect that the number of reps my body is able to push out will be reduced, if only for the first few sessions.

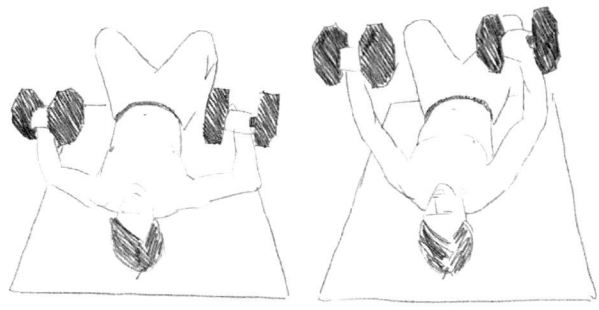

[figure26]

For the chest, I do two different exercises, a basic chest press (figure 26) and a butterfly press (figure 27). Although every other human I have ever seen does these lying down on a weight bench, I have always preferred to do them lying directly on the floor, as I feel better supported and do not require a spotter.

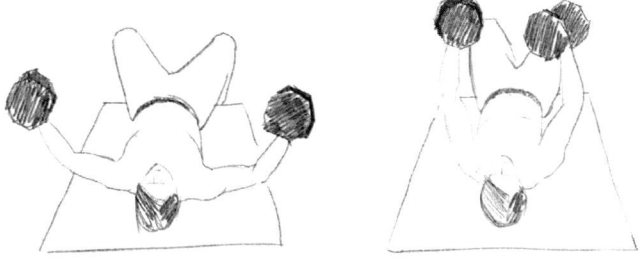

[figure27]

In the beginning, I lie on my back and hold my hands outstretched in front of me, palms up, as if I had a straight bar perched upon them. I allow my hands to drop slowly down until they are just to either side of my chest. I then push them back up to the starting position, remembering to end with my elbows slightly bent (not locked), to ensure my muscles remain engaged throughout the motion. When strong enough, I do a pinch-and-hold between my pectorals, aka pecs (figure 28), at the pinnacle of this movement, to help isolate them—which becomes easier to do later, when I add dumbbells in each hand. I often visualize chest presses as upside-down push-ups because it helps me keep my hands a consistent distance apart.

87

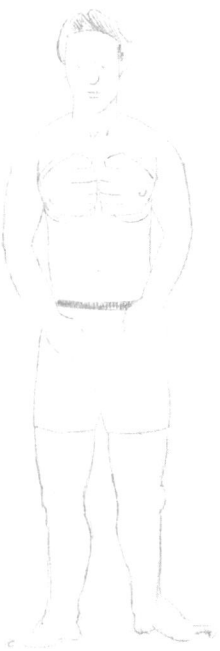

[figure28]

I took a year of judo from a remarkably fit old man when I was in junior high, and he told me to be careful not to build my pecs too much or they would certainly become saggy tits when I got old. He reminded me that they are already the largest muscle group in my upper body and so are easy to grow. I have come to appreciate this bit of advice more and more as the years have gone by, keeping my weights lower and reps higher than is my natural inclination.

I begin butterfly presses lying on my back with my hands up, above my chest, and elbows slightly bent, like I am hugging someone just a little too big around for my hands to come together behind them. I keep my hands in loose fists, knuckles facing one another, and allow them to trace out an arc while dropping slowly down to my sides—maintaining the same slightly bent elbow—until my upper arms nearly touch the floor. I push them slowly back up to the starting position, retracing the same arc and doing a pinch-and-hold between the pecs before dropping down for the next rep. I often think, as I am doing this exercise, that I must look like a real-life action figure, retracting my arms mechanically in anticipation of a spring-loaded bear-hug move. I add dumb-bells in each hand when I feel able.

Although I am aware that my choice to do butterfly presses from the floor prevents me from achieving quite a full range of motion, it is unfortunately a price I must pay to get them done at all, with my many shoulder injuries and a schedule that does not provide for a partner to spot me. This is one small example of doing whatever it takes to adapt my workouts to my life, so as not to *I can't* my way out of getting them done at all.

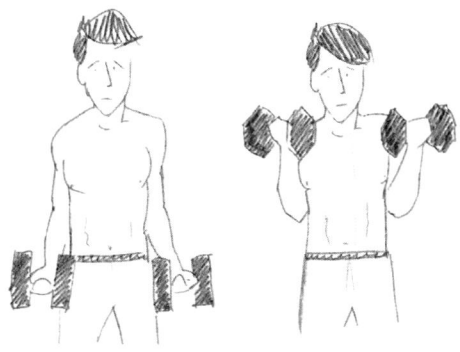

[figure29]

Biceps are best isolated with a curl, and I do two variations. In the first, my weighted hands curl straight out in front of me and may be done from a standing position (figure 29) when starting out or when weights are small. After weights become large, I sit and prop my elbow on my thigh to prevent momentum from dominating the motion. I do the second variation of curls to the inside (figure 30) because the real-life biceps activities I find myself doing often incorporate a bit of both orientations, and I want to be thoroughly strong to accomplish them when the need arises. In either version, I count for each flex-and-hold of the biceps.

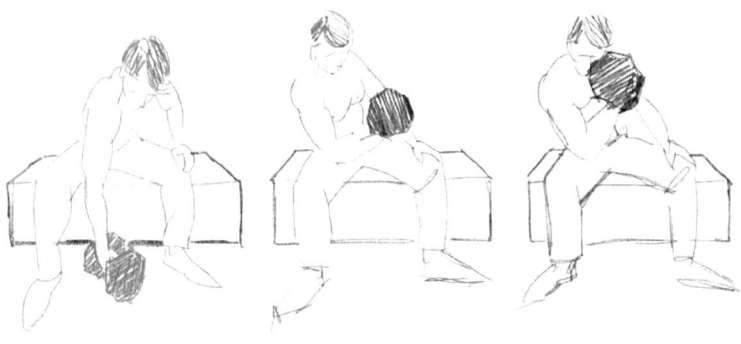

[figure30]

In the first variation, I sit on a chair or bench, with my back straight and feet out in front of me, at about shoulder-width apart. In the beginning, I make a loose fist with my right hand and rest my right elbow on my right thigh wherever it feels most comfortable. Beginning with my elbow bent and fist up, I let gravity provide the resistance, slowly allowing my fist to drop down until my forearm is roughly horizontal, with an angle at the elbow of about 90 degrees. I then bring it back up to the starting position in a slow and controlled manner, flexing my biceps for a moment at the top before doing my next rep. I look directly at it, to intensify focus and maintain conscious engagement, throughout the entire motion. Then I switch and do the same on the left side. This serves as ample practice for when my strength increases enough to add a dumbbell, which requires constant engagement just to keep my grip on it. Because the weight of my fist provides the resistance when I am not yet strong, the addition of dumbbells prompts the motion to reverse, now beginning in the lowered position and ending in the flex at the top.

Even after my first set of these—still with no weight at all—I may be quite sore the following day, depending on my intensity level and number of reps. This illustrates how much applying my conscious focus and intention enhances my body's ability to perform. Although it works particularly well for the biceps—because they are right in front of me while I work them—I make a sincere attempt to consciously channel all of my attention into every muscle I intend to isolate, with each and every motion, for my entire routine.

Biceps, being a very concentrated muscle, grow quickly, making them a good model for me to elaborate on how my numbers of reps go as I gradually build in weight. When I first feel strong enough to add a weight for resistance, I begin with a small weight—like a three- or five-pounder—but even something as mundane as a rock or an empty drinking glass works when it has to. If I am unable to lift it to the starting position, then I accept that I am not yet ready to advance and instead go back to doing it without them and increasing my focus and number of reps over time, until I do feel able to add the weight. When I can lift it proficiently, then I begin with whatever number of reps I feel able to do—usually something like five or eight, although this is based only on personal preference. Until I have built up some overall strength in my body through many consecutive workouts, my energy wanes with each set, so my numbers also decline in each subsequent set of that same exercise.

For my next workout, I attempt to gain in numbers over my previous one, if only by one or two reps per set. With big muscle groups—like biceps and pecs—I tend to feel ready to increase the size of my weight when I am capable of completing about 15 reps, and with small groups—like forearms and trapezius (shrugs)—it is usually more like 25. These numbers are arbitrary to anyone else, since they are what my body tells me is appropriate for it and are bound to vary greatly across the diverse spectrum of human body shapes and sizes.

Since numbers of reps and sets will vary greatly among individuals, I try not to get too hung up on the numbers themselves. Instead, I like to think of them as being like the degrees on a thermometer, which may tell me the precise temperatures of a range my body might perceive to be warm or cold but do not change that perception in any way, shape, or form. They are merely a reference point from which to monitor my performance as it develops.

Muscle endurance develops by doing activities that are light in resistance many times, and muscle strength develops by pushing against heavy resistance just a few times. In this way, numbers allow me to build my body in just the way I feel it should be, so it may be most functionally efficient in my life. If I feel the need to bulk up, I increase weight and decrease reps, and if I am ready to slim down, I decrease weight and increase reps. To extend the same line of thought to my daily life, bulking up means choosing physical tasks that require heavy lifting a few times, like moving furniture or wheelbarrow work, whereas activities requiring only light resistance but many times, like swimming or bicycling, trim and tighten up my body.

My second set of curls is inward, with my feet set farther apart, toes pointed out and knees apart, to make room between them for my hand to trace out its upward arc as I use the inside of my thigh to support the back of my elbow. Again, in the beginning I start with my fist up, slowly dropping it until the angle at the elbow is about 90 degrees, then bringing it back up to a pinch-and-hold, never disengaging the biceps. As with the straight-out variation, I eventually add dumbbells and gradually increase in reps and weight over time, reversing my starting position with the addition of weight.

While doing curls, I vividly imagine that I am focused on pulling Eleanor or one of my kids up from a ledge, where I have come to find them hanging over certain doom. Used to be, if I felt weak, it would be my smaller, younger son, and if I felt strong, it would be Eleanor, but now that the kids are all adult-sized, I just rotate them to keep it feeling fresh.

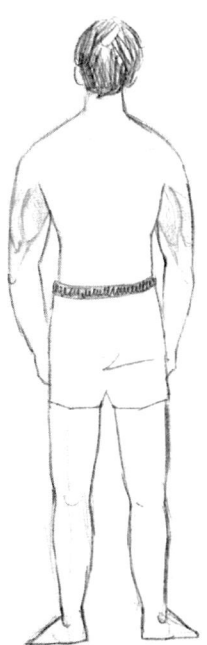

[figure31]

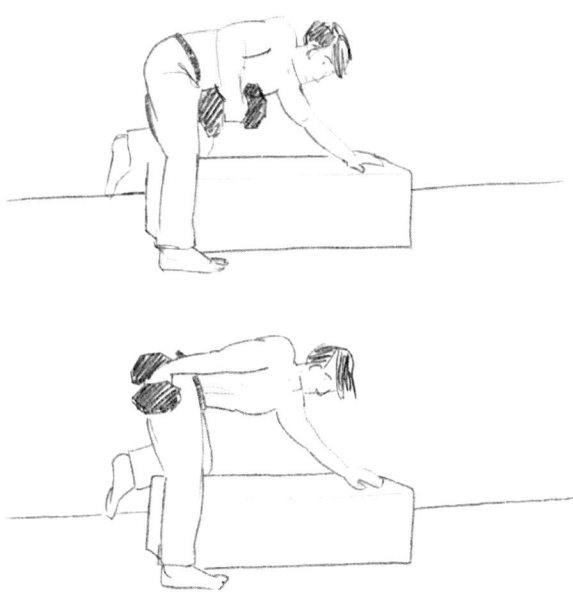

[figure32]

Although there are many good exercises for triceps (figure 31), I like kickbacks (figure 32) the most because they allow a more focused isolation than
any other and may be done even when I am weak. First, I find a bench or two
chairs side by side—anything unyielding and long enough for me to place a
hand and a knee from the same side of my body down, so my torso is approx-
imately horizontal. Even a chair and an end table of reasonably similar height
would work, or, if I should find myself alone in the wilderness with nothing
else, I could just use a log or a couple of boulders.

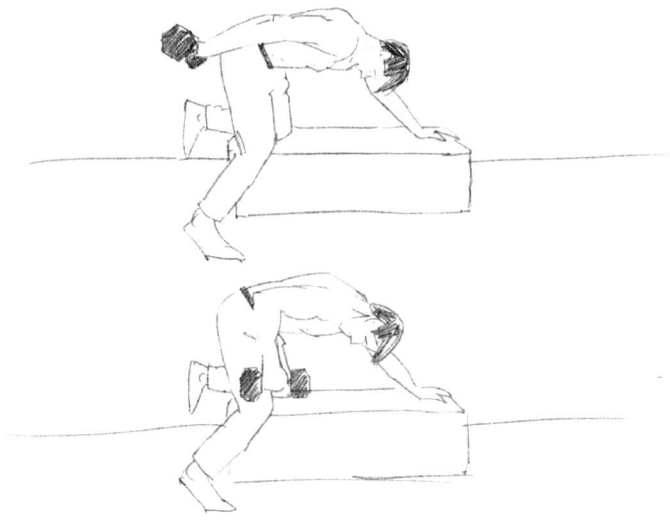

[figure33]

I plant my other foot on the floor, such that it is about shoulder-width from
my planted knee on the other side. I allow my free arm to hang straight down
toward the ground, then raise my elbow toward the ceiling until my upper
arm is horizontal but my forearm and hand are still hanging down toward the
ground. I flex the triceps and slowly trace out an arc—up and back—with my
hand, until my forearm is horizontal as well and my elbow is straight but not
locked. I hold there for a moment, then slowly bring my hand back down to
starting position, keeping my triceps engaged throughout the entire motion. I
do as many as I can and then switch sides and match that number. When I feel
strong enough, I add a dumbbell, and when I am ready for some more intense

isolation, I rotate my wrist as I do each rep, so I begin in the normal position but end with my wrist facing up toward the ceiling (figure 33). I then rotate my forearm back to its starting position (facing my body) as I allow it to drop back down again.

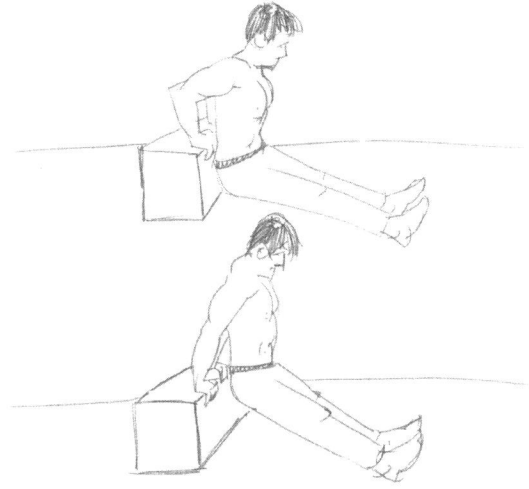

[figure34]

Before my last bad shoulder injury, I would also do a set of tricep dips (figure 34), and when I was younger and just absolutely brimming over with energy, I would add in a set of overhead tricep extensions as well (figure 35).

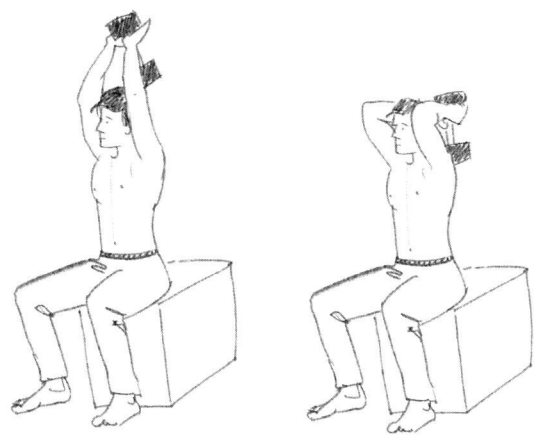

[figure35]

Lats, or latissimus dorsi muscles (figure 36), are best worked with lat rows (figure 37), which begin from the same position as tricep kickbacks but entail lifting my hand straight up toward my torso, as if my elbow were being tugged up by a puppet string, rather than tracing out an arc.

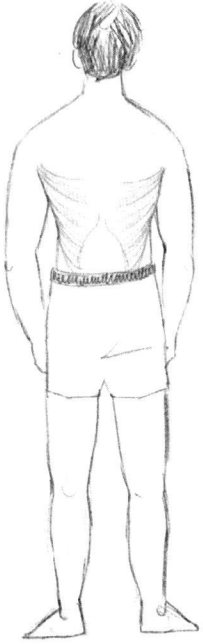

[figure36]

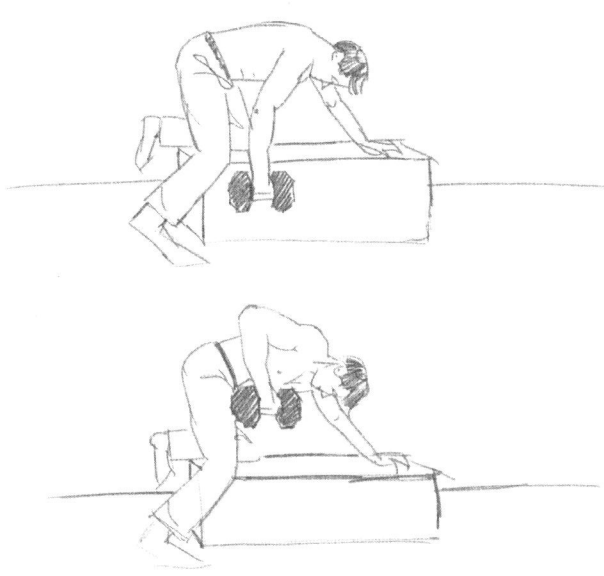

[figure37]

One time, a couple of summers ago, I was working on a little 18-foot Seaswirl boat and had taken it out on the water for a test run after a bit of work, but the motor died and would not start again. Knowing the fee for a tow would be exorbitant even though I was probably less than two miles from the dock, I grabbed my single paddle, straddled the bow, and rowed the boat back against the river current. Now I have a 26-foot boat and lat rows seem easy because I know my vivid imagination is helping to prepare my body for the day I will have to paddle it out of some ridiculous future danger.

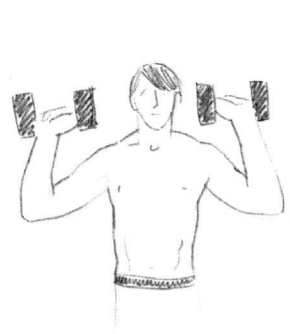
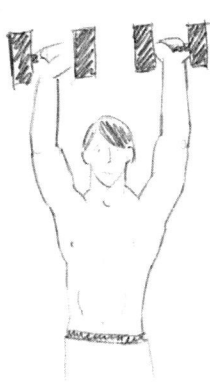

[figure38]

97

I hesitate to mention military presses (figure 38) because I have struggled my whole life to adapt a version of them that does not strain my lower back but gave up years ago. They are an integrative variation for triceps and shoulders, and the only real-life activities I have discovered that emulate them—pushing upward against a torque wrench while mechanicking from my back, and lifting heavy objects overhead to carry or shelve them—also have a tendency to strain my lower back. When I was young, I did military presses aggressively anyway, since the extreme vigor of youth allowed me to power unflinchingly through so much discomfort and my body healed so quickly then. Not to mention, I was not yet in tune with my body enough to discern between muscle-building pain and muscle-damaging pain.

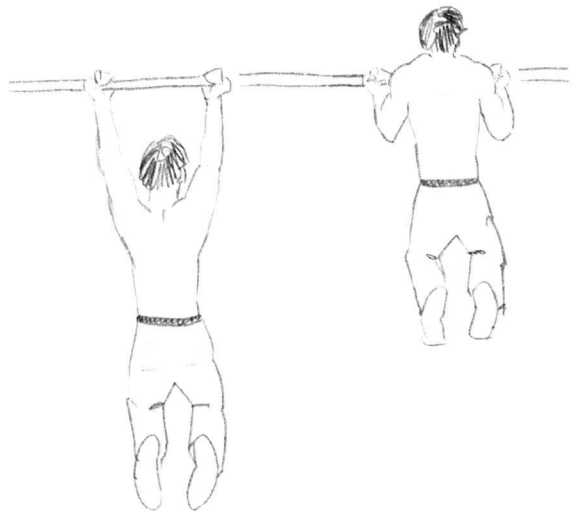

[figure39]

Pull-ups (figure 39) are my last exercise and are dependent on access to a hanging bar or at least a door jamb with a sizable enough edge on its upper border from which to hang by my fingertips. I prefer to do a different variation each session, from gripping at shoulder-width to wide-grip and from an inside grip (aka chin-ups), with wrists facing me, to an outside grip, with wrists facing away (figure 40). For intensity's sake, I imagine vividly that *I* am now the one hanging from the edge of a cliff over certain doom.

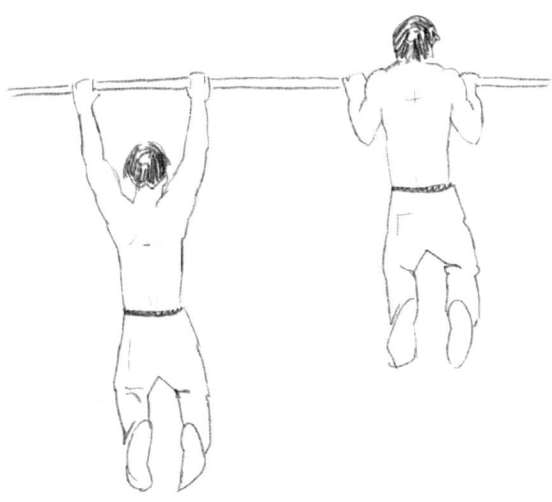

[figure40]

I have lived in many houses and apartments wherein the means to do pull-ups simply did not exist, in which case I would keep in the back of my head that this set was missing from my routine. I would instead do them randomly, as I found myself passing a playground, the perfect door jamb at my friend's house, just the right tree branch, or anywhere else I might knock them out quickly, in passing.

After joining me in my workouts for a couple of years, Zakai had a conversation with his mom about the experience and asked her, "What about cardio?!?"

"Are you kidding?" she asked quite seriously. "You've seen the way he lives. The rest of his *life* is cardio!!" And I like to keep it that way.

CHAPTER 5
Reflections on the Workout

I was born into poverty and did not learn my way out of it until my mid-30s, leading me to develop an adult workout routine independent of a gym membership. After spending a lot of time observing the humans around me managing their own workouts, I realized that choosing to believe a gym membership is a precursor to maintaining a regular workout is a setup for declining vigor if—for whatever reason—a gym, or the membership to it, should become inaccessible.

A set of dumbbells is all I really need to get a good workout, or even two threaded dumbbell handles with a decent collection of disc weights. Actually, even those are not absolutely necessary because they are, in point of fact, just very specifically shaped weights themselves. Which is to say, rocks work fine too, or bricks, or any relatively heavy object for that matter, so long as I may figure a technique for lifting it in the various ways intended.

When I was young, the spontaneously errant nature of my life prevented me from carrying around a weight set, so I simply did lots of calisthenics. Once, during one of the more dramatic times of my youth, I spent 23 days alone in a cell, in which time I discovered that my body is relatively heavy and may be used as resistance for many exercises, although it does require a bit of additional thought. I have, for six months, been limited to a narrow section of wooden balcony—only just long enough to accommodate my fully outstretched body— forcing me to adopt a greatly streamlined routine. I subjected my body to chronic scabbing on my tailbone for years, from the friction of crunches, until I figured out how to protect it with a folded article of clothing tucked underneath.

The reality is, nothing stops me from regularly working out except myself, and any excuse that could be found to avoid doing it is only a surmountable hurdle, challenging me to prove to myself that *I can*. All I have to do is decide whether or not I want it badly enough to push aside all of those good reasons why *I can't* and just *do it*. Doing what I can is so much better than doing nothing at all.

I once read an incredible true story of survival in a *Reader's Digest* magazine. This was way back when it was still well known as an invaluable resource for useful and stimulating reading material, long before the internet lost the publication in a sea of obscure informational tidbits.

It was about a teenage boy, living with his family in deep-country Alaska, who found himself suddenly buried alive in an avalanche while snowshoeing home from school one day with his older brother. He stayed alive for 13 days by systematically flexing each and every muscle in his body over and over again— for all of his waking hours—to keep his metabolism and circulation moving and maintain muscle tone to be ready, should any opportunity for escape present itself. As his ice cocoon enlarged, bit by bit, he first advanced from just flexing to raising each part of his body over and over, then slowly increased his range of motion as it melted out. In the end, he devised a signal to the surface, and his brother saw it and saved him, long after everyone else had given up the search.

For my intents and purposes, the moral of this story is that no matter what resources I have to work with, I should be thankful enough to make the most of them because I may always come to have less. Giving up is an act reserved for my dying moment and certainly not something I would do simply because I felt I did not get a lucky enough roll of the dice on any given day.

The boy buried in the avalanche acknowledged that hypothermia could kill off any part of him if he did not continue making the most of what he had to work with, and he did, indeed, lose a couple of toes to frostbite in the experience. Everything in this life is what we make of it, so I make it a point to be aware of and utilize whatever means I *do* have in every given moment.

Bringing it back around to the workout again, when beginning from a zero point, my second and third workouts will always be the hardest because soreness is at its most intense and my body is weak from a lack of tolerance to muscle-building. At these times, I will decrease both my numbers and my range of motion until my body recovers, so I may not rebound to the levels of my first workout for several sessions. Making myself go through my routine—even when it is hardest, like on the second one back or on those days when I am just not feeling it—is the very essence of self-discipline because if I cannot make myself do it when I least want to, I will definitely not be able to make myself do it at any other time either.

Imagining myself as the me of 30 minutes from now who has just finished working out and is taking a moment to reflect back upon the present me helps me to take the steps, one by one, necessary to go from one to the other. I feel like I have already done it, so now going through the process of doing it seems only the completion of *what is*, coming full circle.

Music is a seemingly small variable with an enormous influence on my routine in its ability to alter my attitude toward the task at hand. I listen to many different genres, depending on the time of day and my particular mood in the moments I come to fit in my workout. I most often find myself listening to aggressive music, because this 30-minute period every other day is sometimes my only chance to physically push out all of the pent-up aggression I have built up during the couple of days' worth of waking hours leading up to it. Variety is the spice of life, so I vary my music widely and frequently, and I find pros and cons to every genre. After taking two terms of hip-hop dance class in college— in hopes of one day taking my graceful wife out dancing without embarrassing her entirely—I gained a new appreciation for music that carries a strong beat, which I couldn't even discern in music before.

Music also seems to occupy some amount of my conscious focus budget— or desktop memory, as Eleanor likes to call it—such that my body's innate desire to follow the beat takes away some degree of what would otherwise be a more focused hold with each rep. When I work out in silence, I feel much more focused and concise—less distracted from my here and now. Because I am not thinking about a beat, a song's overall message, or any other of the many ponderings these may lead me to, I am all business, knocking out one exercise after another, with little or no pause between. I prefer to workout to music, but, for the stimulation of variety, I tend to alternate this as well.

Between the auditory distraction of music and my own vivid imagination running wild through so many repetitive sets, keeping count of my reps has become difficult over the years. I have learned to leverage my imagination by projecting, vividly, a three-dimensional count with my mind's eye as I go. If I should still manage to lose count, then I err on the side of more reps rather than less, so as not to lose any muscle over it.

As the years go by, variety keeps my routine fresh. I play music or not, start with core and finish with upper body or vice versa, go fast or go slow, maybe just scramble up my sets entirely. If I realize afterward that I have forgotten some set, then I begin with it in my next session, since energy overall wanes over the course of the workout.

Time of day also plays an important role in the quality of my workout. I feel working out is much easier at night than in the morning because my body is as limber as it will get all day and my juices are really flowing. In the morning I am stiff and my brain has yet to fully engage my body, so I have to push myself to get through it, and it feels less effective. Eleanor feels her physical energy dwindling as the day goes by, so she is the opposite, preferring morning workouts because she is fresh and crisp then, while night sessions require her to push harder to get through them. Regardless of our particular preferences, learning to listen to our own bodies allows them to optimize their performance. Of course, many days come in which I have only a tight window of time in my day to squeeze in my routine, in which case, I must fall back on my self-discipline to make it happen, despite my preference.

I don't like working out on a full stomach, but I have learned that on the days when I have to—if I am to get a workout in at all—beginning my routine with lifting the bigger weights of upper body first and finishing with core exercises ramps up my metabolism early on, so by the time I get to abdominals, I no longer feel so bloated that I am disinclined to finish.

The *power hour* refers to the 30 minutes before and the 30 minutes after a workout. It is important to know about because it pertains strongly to metabolic momentum. If I sit still all day long, metabolically my body is resting, which means any extra calories—those above what the body needs to break even—are slowly being stockpiled into my fat cells, to be later extracted when my body needs energy but is not intaking food. Working out forces my metabolism to shift to the other direction, immediately burning whatever calories I put in to fuel the work of lifting rather than stocking it away for later, and—with continued exertion—even drawing from fat stored away if I have not consumed enough. Eating within the power hour is far more efficient for our body's metabolic flow, since food is broken down into raw materials for rebuilding itself and the energy needed to fuel those reactions—which it promptly does—instead of being redundantly stored away, only to be broken down again for use later.

When I was younger and yearned to transform my spindly bird-body into a stouter, heartier one, I focused on perpetual caloric intake—primarily during the power hour—as this was my chance to most directly leverage my efforts. If a day should ever come that I find myself desiring to lose weight, I would still strive to eat my largest meals within this timeframe to reduce the amount of fat my body would otherwise be inclined to stockpile. My general preference is to eat something small and protein-rich about 20 minutes before my workout, then reward myself for heavy, calorie-burning exertion with something more voluminous afterward.

I never do two sets that work the same muscle group back-to-back because working a different area in between gives recovery time and a fresher sense of zero point for the next set. By that same token, nearly every muscle group in my body is relaxed while I am doing my best to consciously isolate only the one or ones being worked, therefore I truly have no reason to actively *rest* between sets. Also, this decrease in heart rate and respiration effects a reduction in my metabolic momentum. Herein lies the key to my workout routine requiring only about 30 minutes per session.

Not stopping to rest also allows me to build in mental intensity over the course of my workout, to offset the waning of my physical energy. I dredge up all the suppressed aggression and pent-up angst I have experienced since my last workout to replay as leverage for increasing my degree of intensity. On the rare occasions there have not been any such experiences—of late—I dig deep to find older, more deep-seated anger and frustrations, working hard to push them all out, one workout at a time. Over time I have learned that coming to terms with and pushing out these negative emotions that are associated with difficult past experiences helps me to balance my spiritual self. Not doing so regularly leads me to have more stressed outbursts in my day-to-day life, which I later regret, and which build up in the long term as well.

Doing this has further taught me that conscious control over my body's hormonal secretions is often possible but requires a strong force of will, exercised through self-discipline. In service, I was taught that when crunch-time comes and I get buried too deeply in pending tasks to anticipate them anymore—like a Tetris match on its way to wrapping up—the most efficient solution is *slowing down to go faster*. Being hurried or rushed will only increase the probability that I will make mistakes, which will need to be remedied before moving on, therefore burying myself deeper in impending tasks. Instead, by consciously slowing my breathing and heart rate and focusing on each of my actions being as concise as possible, I may most efficiently dig myself out of this hole. I have to remember to keep perspective and realize that I have the same number of tasks ahead of me regardless of how efficiently (or inefficiently) I handle them. I have also learned to repress my stress response during moments like these by using my mind's eye to see myself from above. I imagine I am seeing myself from farther and farther above, putting into perspective just how insignificant these seemingly intense moments are, relative to all of the other moments transpiring during the same span of time on this giant speck of dust in the middle of cosmic nowhere. In the same way that I use these techniques to reduce the anxiety induced by my adrenal secretions, allowing me to power through such intense moments, exhibiting behaviors that a particular hormone might induce also has a tendency to trigger the secretion of those hormones.

For example, an older male friend recently asked me what I thought about him taking testosterone supplements as a means of overcoming his waning energy level and sex drive. I attempted to guide him to a more natural solution than tinkering with his system's innate balance by pointing out to him that, conversely, if he were to choose to work out harder and be more active—while also choosing to have more ejaculations—this would serve to affect a *natural* increase in his testosterone level. Other commonly known ways to increase testosterone levels naturally include a whole-food diet, sunshine on the skin, plenty of good sleep, and reducing alcohol consumption—some of which my friend had room to improve upon as well.

The unfortunate reality of his situation was that, when he was a young man, his body prioritized the production of testosterone, keeping him edgy and eager for the females. This increased the chances of his reproducing at an age when his sperm had the highest probability of success, both in fertilization and beyond. However, as he aged, his body found its balance with less and less naturally produced testosterone, and because it happened over the course of many years, he had not noticed until awakening one morning to find himself feeling markedly less potent. Had he spent the years since pushing hard in regular workouts and following the other healthy habits that lead to naturally higher testosterone levels, this day might never have come.

Finding my own version of the eye of the tiger, intensity of a steel trap, shark in a guppy tank, or what have you has been important for learning to have conscious control of my own adrenal secretions. Adrenaline is my body's physical manifestation of my mental intensity, so the vividness of my imagination is the key to amplifying or suppressing it. I spend my workouts playing out in my head, vividly, all of the carnal desires of my violent instinctive inclinations, that I may never see them spill over into the rest of my life.

This is also what allows a regular workout routine to be the strongest tool I have for frustration, anger, pain, and stress management. Social constraints already require that I swallow such things in the moment and sweep them under my little mental rug to get through the days. Having them already squirrelled away gives me built-in fuel to gradually feed to my fire through each session. I find myself frequently thanking people like that jerk who held his power over me at the checkout counter, or the supervisor who made me *yessir* them even though I knew they were wrong, for some truly ripping workouts the rest of the week.

Although anger is powerful, for most of us the best amplifier of strength through adrenaline is fear, especially fear for one's very life. This has been demonstrated countless times throughout history by humans performing inconceivable physical feats, saving themselves or their loved ones from certain death. It is also why, when I need a real performance boost, I imagine that my life is actually in danger.

Of course, being always more intense is not sustainable forever. Our genes build in preset developmental checkpoints for our bodies, like at what age our first tooth will grow in or when we will get our first gray hair. They are not set in stone but rather variable, depending on what ingredients we give our bodies to function and develop with and what environmental stimuli we expose them to. I mention this because, with age, my body has gradually changed from being innately flexible, supple, and resilient in youth to a stiffer, more fragile condition in midlife. As far as my genes are concerned, this all revolves around reproduction and my ability to secure a mate and raise offspring while I am still young and cute and healthy enough to do so. As a result, however, expecting my body to continue to build in intensity for its entire existence is not realistic.

My body was most capable, and I was able to push the biggest numbers with it, both in weight and in reps, at age 28. I spent that year focused on constant caloric intake and building—if only a tiny bit every workout—to where I was maintaining ten additional pounds of lean, ripped muscle on my naturally six-foot, 170-pound bird body. Then I got a stomach flu lasting five days, in which time I lost roughly 20 pounds of that hard-earned muscle and then some, leaving my body emaciated. I had only just regained my natural body weight and strength again when I turned 30 and my body began telling me—in earnest—not to push so hard, with the development of a hernia, a stress disorder, and food sensitivities that would later develop into full-blown allergies.

My numbers, in weight and reps, are at their cap for my particular body at its particular age and stage of development. I know this because when I attempt to increase weight, no matter how little, I feel abdominal pressure pushing uncomfortably against my internal hernia mesh patch and my shoulders aching with the pain of slight reinjury, rather than of muscle-building soreness. The sad truth is, I know my numbers are destined to gradually decline as the later years of my life progress, but knowing this prevents me from persistently reinjuring myself as I go through the process. I try to keep in mind that my workout should always be a dynamic reflection of my life, adapting to what happens to me (aging included) and what I want it to be able to do.

For instance, if I am planning a backpacking trip, I do more squats and shrugs to get my body ready in the places I know I will need it. If I am gearing up for a biking event, I go bicycle crunch crazy and become a sudden regular in local spinning classes. When I know I am going to Hawaii to visit family there, I skip the workout entirely for as many laps in the pool as I may muster for the entire week before so I know I will be strong for surfing. Adapting my routine in response to the changes of my life, keeps it conscious and stimulating and prevents my interest and motivation from wavering.

Each of our bodies is a point on a nearly infinite spectrum of different sizes, shapes, and abilities that are each changing every day of our lives, so our workouts should be reflectively unique and dynamic. I have learned to embrace the idea that I do not *have to* do exercises in the orthodox way; rather, I do them as my body tells me it should be doing them, in each workout, on a day-by-day and case-by-case basis.

I do not often find myself in a proper gym with others while running through my routine, yet I have several times overheard personal trainers advising their clients *not* to do particular exercises as they see me do them because it is *wrong*. Approaching fitness in such a way as to insist there is but one *right* technique or method to any motion is certain to exclude a percentage of the population whose bodies are not *currently* capable of doing it in just that way. Doing what *we can* is so much better than doing nothing at all, which is exactly what people are inclined to do when they are told that the only way they are able to do it *is wrong*.

If, at this moment, I am not able to do crunches without letting my shoulders touch the ground between reps, it does not mean I *can't*, it just means I'm currently working up to it—regardless of whether I *ever* get there or not. If my long-term surfing experiences have led me to have a far greater lower-back range of motion when compared with everyone else around me, it does not mean I should, therefore, change my routine in a way that does not feel right to my body. Human bodies vary greatly, and my body is mine to develop as I see fit, for the purposes of whatever life I choose, at any given time.

Over time, I have come to feel like my regular workout is a necessary component to balancing my overall health in all regards: physically, mentally, emotionally, and spiritually. Without it, I quickly begin to feel the pent-up aggression that accompanies suppressed stress and its imbalancing effects on my physiology.

A dog's physiology is at peak performance when it is running trails to hunt and scavenge food daily, like wild coyotes and dingoes still do. Our human bodies are designed to forage and hunt by foot each day, using all of our muscles and brain power to find the calories we need to survive, like the small pockets of remaining primitive humans around the world still do. Since we, as modern civilized humans, do not have to do that anymore, working out on a regular basis, coupled with the increased activity level it drives, helps our bodies to find and balance a more natural caloric budget. Maintaining a regular workout routine drives the flow of metabolic momentum required for each of us to perpetuate our own natural balance of staying healthy.

SECTION 3: FALLING OUT OF HEALTH

Because our macroscopic bodies are the result of a vast multitude of complex microscopic interactions—teeming with countless other microscopic life-forms, each caught in their own struggle for survival—they are prone to fall out of health, regardless of the efficacy of our healthcare strategies or the diligence with which we adhere to them.

CHAPTER 6
Accidents, Injuries, Sickness, and Surgery

None of these events—accidents, injuries, sickness, or surgery—rank highly when considered among life's many experiential offerings, yet none of us remains entirely unscathed of their debilitating and often lasting effects. They are among the prices we must pay for our opportunity to live in this world, and they are tied together by an intense physiological thread.

Pain

I remember hearing Rachel say, in her last year of life, that *life is pain management*. As kids, we were told she had died peacefully in her sleep—which was true, to some extent. My aunt Brandy broke it to me in my late teens that she had actually taken an overdose of sleeping pills because she felt no longer capable of tolerating the pain.

I do not imagine I am alone in feeling like part of the point of my life is to improve upon the lives my parents have lived. I became aware of this in the couple of years following Rachel's death, while grappling with my own depression and trying to figure out how to pull out of it in the long term. I began to tease apart pain itself because I somehow knew this was the key to improving on her view of the world, for my life.

Physical pain is a signal sent from some part of the body to the brain, where it is perceived. It serves the purpose of informing us of some damage or imbalance in our body so we may take action—or cease action—to avoid further damage or imbalance. This applies equally well to the pain experienced in placing one's hand on a hot stove burner as to the muscle pains resulting from a buildup of metabolic waste associated with inactivity.

Our perception of pain intensity is relative, based on the brain's comparison of it to all of the previous pains we have ever perceived before, with emphasis on those we have experienced most recently. As with our perception of hot and cold intensity, it changes as our lives progress. This is the natural process by which we build up tolerances to the damaging effects of our environment, which we must endure as a normal side effect of living.

For this reason, my career server colleagues and I have tolerances to the pain of touching and holding hot plates that wax and wane as a function of how many hours we are putting in. It is also responsible for our ability to become tolerant of other activities—like walking barefoot—that subject our bodies to enough regular damage as to build up calluses on them.

I believe we mostly forget the first few formative years of our lives soon after they have passed because the intensity of pain experienced by our brains through the process of physically hulking out from infancy through toddlerhood is far more extreme than any others our bodies are expected to face for the rest of our lives.

If, at the age of three, we still remembered vividly the pain of growing in a mouth full of teeth and all the growing pains associated with our infantile colic, a stove burner hot enough to burn our hand might hardly make us flinch. Instead, the system resets itself by making us forget all about it, so we begin our post-infancy lives with no pain tolerance at all.

This allows for our pain-avoidance instinct to kick in, preventing us from senselessly maiming our bodies beyond repair, through our most fearless and headstrong next several years of development as we learn from experience (mistake-making). Note that our bodies also have their highest overall resilience and most potent reparative capabilities during this time period.

My experience tells me that our emotional pain system operates in much the same way. We start out gullible and easily trusting but grow to be gradually more guarded as we are continually hurt by the disappointments of our experiences with others or with the universe, trusting in an optimal outcome less and less until we become incrementally jaded. As with physical pain, our most intense emotional injuries of early developmental childhood—the physical breaking apart from the mother, coming to terms with the meaning of the word *no*, and so on—are wiped clean from our memories soon after.

My first conscious memory may well have been sheer pain. I say *may have been* because my early memories are sparse and disjunct, so knowing which one—of the few scattered three-year-old memories I have retained into adulthood—was chronologically first is hard to say. What I can say is that I spent three days of that year at Seattle General Hospital as an inpatient for genital surgery, to be circumcised as a precursor to correcting a birth defect. These are the facts of what occurred, which I was later told by older relatives who were present.

What I remember is screaming awake on an operating table to excruciating pain in my groin, with a young black man in surgeon's scrubs slicing away at my privates. He was almost as caught off guard by the anesthesiologist's mis-dosing as I was and happened to be alone in the room with me when it happened. He yelled frantically over my incessant screaming, "The more you scream the more it hurts, the more you scream the more it hurts!" He held me down until they could inject me with more anesthetic and I passed back out. I also remember a brief and doped-up visit with family in the lobby, but I was brought out on a stretcher, with a little tent over my junk.

My physical pain scale was forever skewed. Later that year, I fell off the roof of a barn Rachel deconstructed for materials to build our cabin back in the woods. It was a 30-foot drop into tall grass, and my lightweight body suffered no damage from the impact except for my left hand, which was sliced to ribbons by a pile of broken glass. This proved to be the beginning of a long and painful life for my unlucky middle finger, which took the brunt of the damage and has since been very nearly amputated or crushed off a further three times.

At five, my left hand was sewn up again after I nearly sliced off the same middle finger pulling myself up onto a school bus stop roof, using a half-broken window. I remember crying because there was so much blood that it freaked me out, but the memory does not include pain.

Shortly thereafter, my mother's death rocked me. I spent a long time wallowing deeply in the pain it caused me before realizing it was my choice to do so and I did not *have to*. I decided that instead of shutting down over it, thereby doing myself the disservice of living a bland and colorless life, I would choose to use my pain to prod me into action, breaking the cycle of depression and beginning me down my lifelong road of building positive associations with pain.

I spent the vast majority of my childhood and adolescence barefoot, and I remember several experiences in which others were not just surprised but in some way concerned that I had no apparent sensitivity to the pain of gravel, thorns, or whatever else might get stuck in my feet. I received similar responses when I moved to Hawaii in my late teens, as I had no qualms about walking barefoot on fresh lava rock or live reef, regardless of how much they might cut me up.

As my life has progressed, I have come to understand that pain marks my brightest experiences, to the extent that when I have no pain anywhere on my body, I feel somewhat numb and certainly less alive. If I am not feeling pain, then what am I feeling? No notable signals to the brain from my body: *null*. Pain gives me something to come up against, and without it, my modern life of walking around, waiting in lines, and sitting in cars to go back and forth to a job—in which I do the same simple tasks over and over again—is not only way too easy to be stimulating, it is rather mundane. Pain makes life challenging and remarkable, and a life entirely without it, to me, would be downright unstimulating.

Although I was never on quite the same frequency as all of the jocks I found myself working out amongst in the high school weight room, their common phrase "no pain, no gain" caused me to have an epiphany about the tie-in between pain and working my body. So long as I could discern the difference between the pain of muscle soreness from building them, and the pain of muscle injury, my level of fitness was a function of how much pain of soreness I could tolerate. This applies equally well to real-world physical labor tasks, as the more work I achieve, the more pain my body endures for it, and the prouder I am of my resulting accomplishments.

I am aware that, among other humans, this perspective earns me the label of masochist, but I am happy to bear it with pride for the benefits it gives me and the amazing feats it allows me to perform.

Now that I have lived beyond the age at which my mother passed, I feel secure in my revision of her belief: life is *not* pain management, rather it is *expectation* management. From my view of it, her insistence on focusing so intently on just *managing* the pain that came her way was her undoing. Had she instead understood that pain was *to be expected*—no matter our particular roll of the dice—and focused her energy instead on channeling it into something, she might still be here today. I am reminded, in relating this idea, of my struggle with cigarettes.

My older sister Stacey gave me my first cigarette when I was nine, and I continued life as a smoker for the next 12 years, until Christmas Day of the year Eleanor was pregnant with Zakai. For the first few years I enjoyed my time as a smoker because I, like the other street rats among whom I was counted, had little or no sense of self-worth and so I did not care about the damage it did to my body. However, after meeting Eleanor and beginning to build care for myself, the habit became something I rued for all of the time and money it lost me and the vigor I chose to forgo.

Every month for the last five or so years that I smoked, I decided at least once to try to give it up. I would diminish my consumption and not buy any more, but my focus on the struggle of *trying* to quit always dominated the forefront of my mind, distracting me from whatever else I might be doing. I found the struggle so difficult that I eventually gave in every time and began bumming singles off my friends until they razzed me into buying myself some more, then the cycle would begin anew.

When Eleanor got pregnant, I knew that for the sake of my own self-worth and to lead a good life as an example for my kids to follow, I had to figure out how to shake off the old smoking habit. I told her this, and we made an agreement that, as of a near future date—which we would mark on the calendar—I would no longer *be a smoker* and that I would instead, from then on, begin a new phase of my life as Colin, the *nonsmoker*.

As a man of my word, making the agreement with her was my way of creating for myself a bound contract. Having it on the calendar for a little while gave me the opportunity to truly appreciate my last few smokes—like I knew they were my last—and also to anticipate and mentally prepare myself for the day that I would awaken as the new me. The struggle of *trying* to quit was no longer a part of the equation.

When the day came, I felt at ease to tell my smoker friends I just did not smoke cigarettes anymore, simple as that. They went about their lives taking smoke breaks, and I proceeded to use that time to be more productive. A little over a week later, after having some drinks, I took a puff off a friend's cigarette, but my body, now being clean of nicotine, recognized it for the toxin it was. I got green in the gills and had to lie down for the rest of the evening, feeling downright sick. I have not smoked a cigarette since.

I am reminded of this experience because Rachel was doing the same thing in focusing so intently on the struggle of *tolerating* her pain, rather than just acknowledging and accepting that pain was *to be expected* so she could go further and figure out some functional coping strategies.

My friend Darryl is fond of the old Buddhist saying "Pain is inevitable; suffering is optional." This is applicable to discomfort as well, since experiences that are uncomfortable need not necessarily be unpleasant. Times of pain or discomfort contrast with times of pleasure or comfort in our lives, and a deep appreciation of the one requires a deep appreciation of the other. In other words: how would we know how much we should appreciate the times we are pleased and comfortable if we have never truly experienced and appreciated the times we are displeased and uncomfortable? Without knowing the stark contrast of these conditions, how are we to truly know the value of either? I consciously appreciate my pains and hardships so I may more thoroughly appreciate my pleasures and ease as well.

Our Self-Healing Biological Machines

From deep underground to the dissipating edge of our atmosphere, planet Earth is teeming with life. Every step we take compresses a mind-boggling array of soil insects, earthworms, and entire microscopic communities, all interacting away before we ever come along and long after we have passed. Beyond breathing out the carbon dioxide that plant life converts back to oxygen for us, we are interacting with countless life-forms in every breath, as a substantial proportion of the "dust" particles in the atmosphere are fungal spores, plant pollen, or bacteria—not to mention all of the exfoliated dead cells floating in the air all around us. That each of us *exists at all* influences every other creature on the planet, in one way or another, before we even think to consider how each of our *actions* affects everything else. This alone makes for another great argument against carelessness.

From a microscopic perspective, our bodies themselves are literally biomes on a scale comparable to the Earth, with a myriad of different ecosystems nested within one another, from our skin right through to our guts. Just like cows, depending on their bacterial populations to digest their primary food source, our survival requires that our microbial populations maintain their diversity and overall health, too.

This idea of immersive biological integration is hard to accept for some humans, who instead choose to perceive themselves as distinctly separate from the ecological interaction web for having lives that unfold entirely in artificial environments of our own creation. We have now grown, however, into the species with the most overt connection to all others as we turn large swaths of the planet into agricultural fields, fill the atmosphere with our collective pollut-ants, and satisfy our craving to hunt and fish for the biggest, strongest, and most healthy *trophies* among our ecological contemporaries.

Because our human species has evolved on planet Earth to fill a particu-lar ecological niche, that of the often nomadic, tribal hunter-gatherer—just as all of the other critters have evolved into their own particular roles—much of my approach to the health of my body is framed from that same naturalist perspective. My healthcare strategy is simply the least invasive and most natu-rally empowering, with a conscious eye toward prevention, and my faith in this approach is anchored by the instinctive satisfactions I feel while running trails barefoot with my kids or sitting around a campfire with my dogs, watching it burn down late into the night.

My son Zakai likes to point out to me that although our bodies were evolved in the context of a wild planet Earth, all of the materials we have pulled from the planet to create our own artificial environments have still come from nature. He goes on to say that everything we create—even to the extent of novel chemical compounds—are put together from natural ingredients. Since we came from nature to begin with, he concludes that everything we perceive to be artificial in our world is actually natural at its core as well. I admit that he is not wrong. However, since the wilderness in which our bodies evolved is still intact in many places in the world, it would obviously be a more optimal habitat for our human organism, given the alternative of our modern civilizations.

Our bodies were not made to sit around day after day watching television, playing video games, and binging on junk food, so it is no wonder they would respond adversely to such conditions. Our modern-day human bodies now live much like the animals studied by biologists, existing in comparatively ster-ile, walled containment units. Admittedly, we are walled in with an unending variety of toys and gadgets intended for stimulation, but between the lack of real-world objects to see within our clean geometric buildings and the energy we no longer expend to hunt and gather, our populations are riddled with a variety of unhealthy neurotic tendencies and stress disorders.

I am reminded of the bears I saw in the zoos of my childhood, long before the humans entrusted with their care gave any thought whatsoever to their comfort, pacing nervously back and forth within their entirely concrete enclosures, snapping periodically at the hordes of gawking onlookers. They exhibited none of their natural behaviors because they lacked the natural stimulations of their intended environment, just like us.

We humans even go a step further from our innate tendencies, as so many of our behaviors are now in response to the social pressures imposed on us by the other humans around us. I feel a vast majority of humans would be hard-pressed to say just what it is they are naturally inclined to do, given all of the social conditioning beginning in our families, right from birth.

Having little to no social expectations during my formative years allowed me to discover many of my own instinctive tendencies. For as long as I can remember, I have been highly averse to having my nails clipped, and as a young child I avoided it with tenacity. Thankfully, Eleanor introduced me to the practice of filing them instead, which has come as some relief to me. Wearing clothing feels encumbering to me, so the less I may get away with wearing, the more content I am. This leads into my inclination toward warmer weather and warmer locations in general. Left to my own devices, I am inclined to bathe properly only every three to four days, although I love to take periodic rinses in oceans, streams, or other natural bodies of water—even several times daily, if I am able. I am disinclined to wear chemicals on my skin or hair, be it deodorant, sunscreen, hair gel, or even conditioner, as I am disturbingly conscious of their residues soaking into my body.

However, for the comfort of the other humans around me, I do an assortment of things that go against my own inclinations, from bathing and cutting my hair regularly to wearing body coverings and applying various chemical substances—including deodorant. I am willing to exhibit even more unnatural behaviors that I would otherwise have no interest in, out of sincere gratitude toward my loving wife for all of her unwavering acceptance, even so far as to periodically apply hand lotion and try wearing underwear. Although I am aware that I exhibit many behaviors that may not be optimal for me either physically or spiritually, at the end of the day I feel they are all necessary evils if I am to best tiptoe the fine line between being as healthy as I may be and being as fulfilled as I may be.

If we are to achieve and maintain good health, then we must learn to reawaken our built-in instincts, listen to our bodies, hear what they are telling us, and modify our behaviors appropriately. Our bodies are literally self-healing biological machines in which our souls travel the universe, and as such, they come with a set of pre-programmed behaviors intended to allow our care for them to be innate, even second-nature. That is why our bodies have so many autopilot behaviors that are also within our conscious control, like breathing, blinking, eating, defecation and excretion, the fight or flight response, reflexes like flinching and pain aversion responses, and so many more. Instincts go so far as to pre-program our bodies with specific preferences in diet, sleep schedule, climate, and even such complex predilections as the scent of potential mates.

As an example, blinking at the natural rate each of our bodies requires happens subconsciously, without us having to think about it, but if need be, we may at any time take the controls and shutter our eyes at will. When a situation arises in which an object comes quickly near our eyes, the subconscious takes momentary control to close them instinctively—quickly and tightly—as a means of making the body's self-preservation automatic. But then, some of our lives lead us to get contact lenses, and we use our willpower and self-discipline to overcome the flinch instinct.

Unfortunately, we have now learned to suppress so many instincts that much of our bodies' responses to the happenings of our lives have become downright mysterious to us. Through over-analyzation and the hyper-awareness that we may choose to do whatever we want regardless of what the body tells us, we have become so unaware of our bodies' signals that many of us feel incapable of deducing what may be wrong, much less how to make it right.

Our bodies are designed to maintain their own balance and optimal health, given proper nutrition and a conscious pilot (the self) who is listening and paying attention to its signals and modifying behavior appropriately in response to any shifts out of balance. If we are not giving it enough food or water, it sends us a hunger or thirst signal. If we are working it too hard, it sends us a signal that it is tired and needs a rest, and if we are not physically doing enough, it sends us a signal of restlessness to prod us into action. When we damage it somewhere, it sends us pain signals so we will know from where to remove foreign debris or treat it sensitively thereafter, allowing it to repair and encouraging us to avoid further damaging it. This self-healing property is why we commonly say, "time heals *all* wounds."

Time Heals All Wounds

This truism is obvious with scratches, scrapes, and bruises, but it applies equally well to a whole lot of pretty serious injuries.

Flesh wounds heal just fine on their own, even sizable ones. Although they may result in some temporary imbalances while they draw on the resources of surrounding tissues to make repairs, given time, the body finds its balance again, after healing back to functionality.

My body has healed from a lot of flesh wounds over the course of my life, from the road rash of falling off or jumping out of moving vehicles to bicycle, moped, and skateboard accidents to power tool and construction accidents to injuries sustained performing senseless thrill-seeking activities and silly people tricks. These are all in addition to the self-mutilation I have subjected it to from the slips, trips, and falls of an extremely clumsy youth (when I didn't know I couldn't see) and all of the countless burns and cuts of a lifetime of avid home cooking, supplemented by a few years of professional cooking.

The week before my 21st birthday, I gave myself one of the worst flesh wounds I have ever had, while living in Hawaii and driving around an old 1970s moped that looked like a mini chopper. The motor had no cover on it, so when it got hot, I had to be careful not to touch it. I had just come home from driving it halfway across the island and back and was walking it into the back yard, where I parked it. While opening the gate with one hand, I had to turn the moped sharply toward myself, after pushing it uphill to the back yard.

Unfortunately, I had on flip-flops, and my left foot caught the edge of the concrete walkway, causing me to lose my balance and fall backward (downhill), pulling the moped over onto myself. It would not have been too bad except that the hot motor pinned my left foot to the pavement, searing and scraping the top right off of it. The knobby round bone on the ridge of my foot was a grotesque silver-dollar sized white protrusion, and I could feel that the tendons that had been attached to either side of it were no longer.

I was not insured, and I knew that even if I could somehow conjure up the most experienced reconstructive surgeon ever, my foot could not be remade as it was, and nothing they could do would prevent me from experiencing all the pain of recovery and the future pain of having an old injury of this magnitude. Were I to have taken it to the emergency room, they would have cleaned it up, dressed it, and sent me on my way with a recommendation to stay off it and some strong painkillers. I saw no good reason to go, instead cleaning it up and letting my body heal itself, while carrying on about my normal business to distract myself from the pain. With time, it healed, and although it was sore after long walks for a couple of years and I now wear half a size bigger shoe on that foot, it has otherwise not affected my life whatsoever.

I have an unlucky toe on my right foot (the big one) that has sustained multiple flesh wounds, beginning when I was 17 and dropped a 35-pound Olympic disc weight on it while working out barefoot. The nail turned black and, several days later, was torn off at a raging teenage party, presumably by a passing shoe as I was, of course, barefoot. It took with it a chunk of under-nail flesh, so when it grew back, there was such a big bow in it that I have forever since had a built-in stash spot for something nearly dime-sized. From then on, it has always been my unlucky toe, attracting injuries chronically, having heavy objects dropped or set on it, and being persistently stubbed or scraped.

Several years later, Eleanor was pregnant with Taj and we were living in a little Honolulu apartment with slick vinyl sheet flooring. While shuffling furniture around the apartment, I had my back to a wall and pulled the couch toward myself, not expecting the slick flooring to make it slide so easily. As I pulled hard, up and toward myself, the bottom edge of the couch grazed the top of the bow in my unlucky toenail, tearing it two thirds of the way off.

I did have health insurance at the time and decided to take it to a doctor and see what they might do about it. However, the only time I could get in to see the doctor my insurance covered was in conflict with a checkup appointment for toddling Zakai at another hospital across town. I dropped him and Eleanor off for his appointment and rushed off to mine, hoping it would all work itself out.

I had a pretty long wait, unfortunately, so by the time I got in to see the doctor, he had only enough time to lay out my options: he could inject anesthetic at the tip of my toe and wait 30 minutes for it to reach the base, then tear it off with some fancy medical pliers, or he could insert the needle at the tip of the toe and drive it all the way down to the base before injecting, so I would only have to wait 10 minutes before letting him tear it off, or I could just hold my breath, look away, and let him tear it off right away. Just then I received a call on my cell phone from my pregnant wife with toddler son in tow, asking with severe irritation if she could count on me for a ride or if she needed to call herself a cab. I said I would be right there, hung up, held my breath, and looked away while the doctor tore my toenail the rest of the way out. He sent me away with his strongest sample painkillers and a recommendation that, with a pain tolerance like I have, next time I should just take a few shots and do it myself. I agreed.

Many years later, I set my sights on kiteboarding Immigrant Lake in southern Oregon but discovered on arrival that I had forgotten my wetsuit booties. I decided to kite anyway, as it had taken hours to get there, but the shoreline was covered with sandstone and rocks. My solo launch required that my kite drag me through the rocks on my bare heels for a good 20 feet, before I could grab my board and head for the water. In that 20 feet, I had rock splinters embedded throughout the soles of my feet and lost a sizable chunk of flesh from just below my right (unlucky) big toe. I didn't walk very well for a few days, but it all healed itself within a month or so, and I didn't miss a beat for it.

Our bones heal themselves after being broken or bruised, all on their own. I have broken my right thumb and multiple toes and fingers, some more than once. Although I did not go to a doctor to confirm my diagnosis and reset any of them, they all work just fine for me, despite being crooked and gnarled. I have also bruised bones in my shins and feet a few times, which felt serious enough to have been broken, but they also healed themselves up perfectly well.

I fractured my skull in a high-speed downhill bicycle accident when I was 13, and although I was delivered unconscious to the emergency room, without an actual hole or hemorrhaging, all they could do was soak and stretch the skin around the wound, sew it up, and send me on my way. I removed my own stitches a couple of weeks later rather than suffer the rigamarole of another hospital visit.

Even severe cartilage breaks, like a broken nose, heal themselves over time. Three summers ago, I went out eagerly to catch a quick kiteboarding session before work at my normal spot on the Columbia River, just down the hill from my house. Before getting on the water, I cinched down my waist harness around my ribcage, nice and tight like normal, since it comes loose from all the tugging while I ride.

I did one quick lap across the river, to the Washington side, and was on my way back toward my home shore when I caught a big air that got unexpectedly bigger from a gust aloft. It caught me off guard and I over-rotated, landing hard and fast on my side.

When I got up to ride away, I felt my harness dig painfully into my side and kept trying to push it down off my ribcage. Then I realized the pain originated inside my body, so I headed for shore, where, thankfully, a few of my kiting buddies were getting set up to go out. They helped me land my kite and get my harness off, at which point I could already tell I had broken a rib for the sharp pain I felt every time I exhaled too far out. The guys broke down my gear for me while I struggled to my truck and drove myself an hour to the emergency room. I went in telling them that I had just broken a rib, but their attitude was that I could not possibly know for sure since I was not a doctor, so I had better let them do a bunch of tests and then tell *me* what was wrong with *my body*.

I spent roughly five hours allowing them to perform several tests, scans, and X-rays, all the time yelping in sharp pain for the rib I felt literally kink inward when I would straighten up too much or exhale too far out.

I remembered the real skeleton from my high school life science class and the anatomy and physiology classes I took in college, so I knew from what I felt that the tip of my tenth (false) rib had experienced a break from the cartilage joining it to my sternum. This is what gave me the fluttering feeling—as the cartilage actually kinked inward—and I was a little worried it may be poking me in an organ, but at the end of all the tests, the doctor told me I had nothing apparently wrong with me, so I must have only just bruised the muscles of my ribcage.

When I told him what it felt like to me, he condescendingly explained that I might feel whatever I want about it, but his diagnosis would remain the same, unless I *wanted* him to take more X-rays and run more tests to confirm *my opinion*, which he would be happy to do if I was ready to spend more money and time. Even if it *were* broken, he said, they would only wrap it up and advise me to rest in bed for a few days anyway, since there is only so much that may be done about such an injury. In other words, go home and let your body heal itself. I had health insurance at the time but still received a bill for several thousand dollars. For a couple of years, my rib continued to kink with every sneeze, cough, and crunch, but over time it kinked inward and stayed there, so the nub of its bony end now pokes out of my side.

Stretched and torn tendons and ligaments heal themselves back to functional condition as well, given enough time—even if they are never quite as strong again—and continuing to use our bodies eventually strengthens the supporting musculature to pick up whatever slack remains.

I have stretched the ligaments holding my shoulders together (aka separations) several times throughout my life, but the last one on my left shoulder was by far the worst, whether for the intensity of the impact, my body's reduced elasticity from being older, or a bit of both.

We were homeschooling our kids and had a regular weekly meetup at a local park to socialize with other homeschooled kids. The park was in a small valley, and the drive in had a sweeping downhill curve, which I noted had just been freshly asphalted and looked absolutely delicious to skate on. As soon as the family settled into their groups, I grabbed my board from the back of the car and walked up the hill.

Unfortunately, I had spent the previous few weeks skating the new skatepark that had just been built across the street from our apartment and I did not stop to think about how loosely I prefer to have my trucks adjusted when I ride park versus downhill. I realized it shortly into the ride, of course, but was already going too fast to stop, and the speed wobble caused me to fishtail until I bailed headlong into the same roll that had saved me countless injuries in a lifetime of similar falls. This time, however, was different.

I picked myself up, chuckling at the idiocy of my mistake and noticed my left shoulder was in much more pain than the road rash on its surface warranted. I could also see the tip of my collarbone poking out underneath the skin of my shoulder and could feel that a muscle attaching it to something in my back had been badly stretched. Looking over my shoulder, I could see the bone it was attached to protruding from just under my shoulder blade.

I went back to Eleanor—sitting on her blanket, talking with friends—and asked her to please take me to the emergency room, where they cleaned and patched my open wounds and X-rayed my back and shoulder. A doctor sent me out the door a few hours later with my arm in a sling and a referral to a surgeon who, he advised, would do a fine job of cutting into my shoulder with a laser to re-hang it with some metal pins, screws, and straps for me.

I asked him how long we had been treating this type of injury in this way, and he responded that it was still a relatively new technique, developed just a few years back. I asked what people were doing for this injury before we came up with this technique as a follow-up. He said prior to that, we just let the body heal itself as best it would on its own, supplementing with some rehabilitative physical therapy.

When I got home, I began the two-week process of sifting through the accounts—both online and with people I met in my real life—of every human I could find who had done to themselves what I had and the final outcomes of their recovery choices. Most of them had taken their doctor's advice and gone to a surgeon to have the hardware installed, and only just a few had not, choosing only physical therapy instead—mostly in conjunction with a neoprene support brace worn under their daily clothing to keep their shoulder in place.

However, out of all the many cases I investigated, not one of the people who opted for the surgery *ever* regained their full range of motion, some experienced severe arthritic pains in the years that followed, and all incurred the added pain of surgery and recovery. Additionally, many reported complications with their immune systems rejecting the hardware, and nearly all of them required follow-up surgeries to tighten up or remove screws or pins, some as often as annually. The few people who simply allowed their bodies to heal themselves, on the other hand, all reported an eventual return to their full range of motion, albeit with less strength than before. Needless to say, I never did call the surgeon, I regained my full range of motion in less than a year, and although it remains my weaker shoulder, I still push solid weight with it. As an added superpower, I now have an extra inch of reach on that side.

I have also severely hyperextended both of my knees in a kiteboarding accident, a decade or so ago, resulting in substantial damage to the ligaments behind them. My grandmother on my father's side had passed away, spurring a gathering of the family to honor her and our grandfather's wishes to have their ashes scattered together into the middle fork of the Boise River in the tiny town of Atlanta, Idaho. Dane flew out to my place in Oregon, and we made a road trip of it to catch up.

I had only just learned to kiteboard the year before, and although I was not very good yet, I was still very bold about taking every possible opportunity I could create to gain more experience, so I brought my gear with me in hopes of stirring up a session. Unfortunately, come the end of the family stuff, when all that remained was to drive home, no good opportunity had shown itself. I decided to take a chance and attempt my first session riding a river with the wind blowing downstream, a situation generally attempted only by those who are very proficient already or who have a planned pull-out somewhere downwind.

We drove to the Snake River, not far from Mountain Home, just upstream of where the river begins to grow into the CJ Strike Reservoir. I launched upwind of the highway overpass we had come in on, but it only took me a few runs to find myself sucked so far downwind that my kite flew over the traffic driving by.

I knew I had to get out of the water and walk myself back upwind to take another go at it, but the shoreline was thickly lined with eight-foot-high cattails. Unfortunately, I was still a novice, so I did not know to expect the wind to whip violently up over the berm on which the highway had been built. I rode carefully up to the shoreline, trying to figure out what to do, when my kite caught the whip and popped me 12 feet or so up into the air, right over the cattails. I had not learned to jump yet but thought if I could steer my kite back the way I had come, I would perhaps be able to waft back over the water and pull off a reasonably safe landing. I was too aggressive in my steering, however, and instead was flung full force into the cattails, landing hard, feet first, while being pulled strongly downwind. My whole body slapped down, face-first, into the cattails so fast and hard that both of my legs overextended, forcing my knees to momentarily pop the wrong way. Thankfully the immense force tore out all the bolts holding in my bindings, or it would certainly have been worse.

I tried to get up but could not walk, and Dane was still across the river, running to the car to drive over and help me. My kite dragged me face-first through the sagebrush and goat heads for about a hundred feet before I managed to get it landed. Dane packed up my kite and lines, then went back to find my board for me.

My knees rested over the eight-hour drive home, at which point I could hobble myself around, and given a few days of rest, I returned to work, taking it easy for a while. For the next couple of years I slowly regained the ability to crouch and kneel, and now the only adversity I experience as a result is a loud, painful cracking from my knees after kneeling on them for too long. From what I understand—having known many humans who have incurred similar knee injuries and who do participate in mainstream medicine—there is a high likelihood that I ruptured both of my anterior cruciate ligaments (ACL) to the extent that surgery would have been the recommendation.

Even our more sensitive internal tissues recuperate from damage all of their own accord, like my left ear, which sustained severe chemical burns inside some years ago in a mechanicking accident and still serves me fairly well. I have liked machines my whole life, especially cars, and done my own mechanic work, learning entirely by trial and error. I have owned more than 30 cars, and many of them were resurrection jobs, pulled from fields or parking lots where they had spent years in disuse. My first car was the 1961 Ford van that Rachel left when she died, which sat for nine years in the desert on the unused back acreage of my grandfather's pig farm, waiting for me to bring it back to life.

As a young man, I prided myself on keeping whatever most decrepit-look-ing beater I drove around purring like a kitten. Of course, they broke down often, but I did my best to manage it by selecting cars light enough I could push them out of harm's way myself if something should happen, and I more or less reveled in this adventurous nature of my life. Even later, when our toddlers required of us a more reliable vehicle, I still preferred to let that be the family car while I regularly drove around a good project beater to wrench on for my own stimulation. It was during this phase of life that I had a doozy of an accident one afternoon while changing out the fuel filter on my Bronco II.

We were living in an apartment in Sarasota, Florida, at the time, so I was out in the parking lot, under my truck. I was on my back with very little clearance and had to unscrew the filter to get it off, but it was set into the groove of an I-beam in the frame, so when I got it unscrewed, it was also jammed in. I pried at it with a screwdriver to break it loose, and it popped out violently, splashing dirty fuel all over my face. Thankfully, my body's flinch instinct closed my eyes, quickly and tightly, as the dirty gasoline filled up my eye sockets.

I struggled to get out from under the truck, wriggling frantically from side to side to shimmy out, and when I did, I rolled onto my left side to get myself up off the ground. The gas poured from my eye sockets into my left ear, at which point my whole head exploded into an intense, searing pain. A sudden, torrential flash downpour—which is seasonally common there in the afternoons—pummeled me from above.

I groped my way past the bushes and around the building to our apartment—my burning eyes still tightly clenched—amidst buckets of rain barreling down on me. Eleanor heard my distressed shufflings and snortings at the doorstep as I fell into the door trying to find it, and she came out to help me in. The pain in my face and head was so intense, it was more than blinding; it was crippling. She all but carried me into the shower and flushed out my ear and eyes with tea tree oil, which made the pain bearable. I fell into bed, not daring to open my eyes for fear of discovering I was now blind. My body was in shock, and I quickly drifted into a deep, recuperative sleep.

I awoke in the morning, my eyelids red, crispy, and flaking from the chemical burns, but when I opened them, I was greatly relieved to find that they worked fine. My flinch reflex had been fast enough to save me from any permanent damage to my eyes, but I could feel that my left ear was swollen shut inside, and I received no signals whatsoever from it.

Over the next six months, my hearing gradually returned, although I have forever since lost the ability to hear tones any higher than a gym teacher's whistle on that side. When I get a cold or any kind of ear-, nose-, or throat-affecting sickness, sounds coming into that ear become muffled, eventually fading out almost entirely, and I experience quite a lot of tinnitus (ringing) from it the rest of the time.

I did not even think to go to a doctor about this because I could not imagine that any medical solution to the sensitive tissue of my tympanic membrane (eardrum), having sustained severe chemical burns from filthy gasoline, would leave me any better off than simply allowing my body to heal itself as best it could. As a reaffirmation of this, years later I witnessed one of my kiteboarding buddies rupture his eardrum from getting slapped down on the water real hard, and it resealed and healed itself over the course of just a few months.

Out of thanks for Eleanor's efforts on my behalf, I now wear hearing aids, so as not to drive my sweet heroine of a wife out of her ever-loving mind with my persistent misunderstandings. Ten years or so after the accident, our audiologist friend—who gifted me my hearing aids—was blown away at how healthy my left ear still looked inside, considering the damage it had endured.

Nerve tissue recovers itself from damage as well, although in my experience it may result in a long-term intermittent perception of numbness in the region. The nerves of my neck and shoulders have been damaged as a result of the teenage bicycle accident in which I cracked my skull, from all of my many shoulder separations, and from an overconfident, drunken trampoline accident in my mid-20s after I'd taught myself to do standing front and back flips.

The emergency room doctor who patched me up from the bicycle accident said the nerve damage in my neck would heal itself. I went to see a doctor about the nerve damage to the same place on my neck after the trampoline accident years later, and all of their scans and tests also led him to the conclusion it was best to let it heal itself, sending me home with prescriptions for painkillers and muscle relaxers. Now, roughly 15 years after the last of these injuries, I no longer experience any adverse effects at all from them.

The nerve damage in my shoulders, however, has been chronically exacerbated by my activities since, like pulling out big juniper bushes or being tugged erratically on my skateboard by my antsy pitbull suddenly spotting a random squirrel. The subsequent numbness—which often extends all the way to my fingertips—is a symptom I struggle with when riding a bicycle uphill or sitting at a desk to write for more than about ten minutes. This also prevents me sleeping on my sides for too long.

Despite the minor fallout I experience from the many severe injuries I have subjected my body to, I can still say with confidence that time has healed all of them. Whether these wounds healed overtly or were instead buried under the sequential layering of future experiences, allowing me to ignore them, the pain has been effectively eliminated, as I no longer register it consciously.

If It Isn't Broken, Don't Fix It

There are many pain messages sent to our brains requiring us to make only minor or even no behavioral changes. We must all withstand growing pains throughout our development and the pain of breaking in teeth, but their pain signals serve as more of a status report than a call to any particular action.

Similarly, pain signals from muscle soreness resulting from intense activity serve to inform us that we have worked our bodies more than they are used to. If the body's intention in communicating this message to the brain was that we not work it so hard, then this activity would not serve to make our muscles stronger and the rest of our system more tolerant to this higher activity level. We decide to do something arduous, and our bodies inform us that we have exerted them enough to have torn some muscles in the process of making them bigger and stronger. Whether that information prompts us to become soft and intolerant to future stress from inactivity thereafter or to press on even harder—to make ourselves stronger and more resilient—remains our choice.

In the wild environment our bodies were designed to exist in, their activity and calorie budget would not allow us to cease foraging and hunting because we had injured them. They provide us pain signals in hopes that we avoid that area for a while to allow them to heal optimally, even as we carry on with our business. Pressing on is a *natural* requirement, but the only modern human behavior I have seen that demonstrates an understanding of this is the P.E. instructor's advice proffered to students with a minor lower-body injury: *walk it off*.

Flesh wounds scab up and heal themselves, given time, whether we heed the pain signal they send to our brains and avoid touching them or ignore it and keep tearing off the scab. The eventual scar left behind may be more noticeable if it is not allowed to heal nicely under the cover of that first scab, but from the perspective of our lives and the choices we get to make over the course of that time, the outcome is the same.

If my body is able to heal an injury while I keep on living as if nothing happened, then it should be allowed to. The more I let the pain slow me down, the more atrophy and reduced metabolic flow results, making for a longer and more stressful recovery. Reducing respiration, circulation, and metabolism by resting additionally reduces my immune response to any pathogens my body may be faced with during recovery. Physical therapy to recover from a musculoskeletal wound is all good and fine, but its necessity arises only if I am slowed down enough for the area to atrophy in the first place.

"If it isn't broken, don't fix it" has been the primary mantra of my personal healthcare strategy for my entire life, but when I say "broken," what I mean is broken *beyond my body's own capacity to repair it without assistance*, and when I say "fix it," what I mean is *giving my body the most natural and least invasive assistance necessary to enable it to do the repairs itself*. Of course, these terms are relative and have gradually changed over my lifetime, as I have learned just how severe a condition must be before medical assistance is *actually necessary* and then recalibrated every time I have gone in for medical assistance, only to have them clean it up and send me on my way to let it heal itself. Much to my loving wife's chagrin, as our lives have unfurled, I have required that the ailments of my body be progressively worse before being convinced to take it to the medical industry for assistance.

Meanwhile, I have observed a lifetime of humans around me going to the doctor for every little discomfort, even ones they admit might just be imagined. They seek answers for the anomalous pains and unusual behaviors of their bodies—often of the *status report* variety to begin with—and their doctors humor them with unending prescriptions for laboratory-derived painkillers, antibiotics, steroids, or whatever other new concoction is all the rage, which throw their bodies further out of balance from their naturally healthy state. Even the replacement of hips and other body parts may now be done rather casually, on the simple proclamation of pain.

Most of the humans I have known who avidly take their bodies to the doctor to be *fixed*, under the perceived pretense that pain or discomfort means they are in some way broken, tend to perpetuate their own perception through all of the drugs and other treatments advised by said doctor. In most cases I have witnessed, this process is not the means to any particular end but rather a neurotic behavior exhibited by both doctor and patient, often resulting in a far more complicated picture and overall worse health than existed in the first place. A persistent belief that something is wrong with our bodies leads them to manifest this expectation, just as they will reflect the expectation that they be healthy and strong.

Shortly before meeting Eleanor, I had a brief relationship with a woman who treated her health in this way, which resulted in my daughter, Adriana, being born. Unfortunately, I spent Adriana's first few years of life battling in court with her mother to be granted visitation and was court-ordered—for six months—to have my visits with her be only at her mother's home and under supervision. Of course, this led me to make many in-person parenting decisions based on the expectations and beliefs of her mother, rather than my own, for fear of losing visitation rights altogether.

One night during this time, I received a late-night phone call from Adriana's mother, who was distressed over Adriana's physical condition. Apparently, she had a severe tummy ache, which—her mother reported—had become common recently and had resulted in late-night visits to the emergency room all week. She had called me out of frustration, insisting I come pick Adriana up and take her in, as she was tired of doing it herself and expected I would share the responsibility of what she perceived to be our daughter's *needs*. Although I did not agree this was a need, nor that it was even in her best interest, I complied because I did not want to lose the ground I had gained in court.

When I picked her up, she seemed fine. I asked about her tummy on the way to the emergency room, and she became suddenly stricken by it, doubling over and groaning in apparent pain. A few minutes later, as we pulled into the hospital, she had completely forgotten it and again seemed without ailment.

To me, this was an obvious drama behavior, successfully performed to gain the attention and concern of her mother, which now forced me to go against my own better judgment to avoid her mother's attempts to prove me an uncaring parent.

I brought her in to a bored emergency room staff who already knew her by name and obviously understood my role there even better than I did myself. They proceeded to put her through a series of tests and procedures, telling me at the end of each that it had revealed nothing concerning or was simply inconclusive and then briefing me on the next one in line. It became painfully clear to me at about 3 a.m.—just after my three-year-old received a barium enema and a colonoscopy—that the doctor was entirely aware there was nothing wrong with her but was perfectly comfortable subjecting her to whatever he could convince me of, to milk insurance money out of the situation. Now I understood the eagerness with which they had received us, since she came equipped with fully state-funded health insurance, and they knew it from their previous nights dancing the same dance with her mother.

Needless to say, when the doctor approached me to relay the latest news in inconclusiveness and sell me on the next—even more invasive—procedure, I snatched up my daughter, read him off, and stormed out angrily. Her mother, upon receiving her back, clearly understood everything that had transpired without requiring even one single word of explanation, making it quite obvious to me that this was now an established habit for her.

This experience taught me not to go—nor to take anyone I know—to the hospital for anything less than life-threatening injuries or illness, lest the humans running our capitalist-driven medical system create additional health complications in their desire to feed their egos and make money for themselves or the companies they represent. Generally speaking, tummy aches, headaches, and the random aches and pains of the body justify no more action than a conscious consideration of the body's basic needs and a revision in behavior to calibrate and adjust for imbalance—certainly *not* a trip to the emergency room.

Relinquishing my body to our medical system under such circumstances is a loud and clear declaration that I am afraid and uncertain enough how to proceed that I would be willing to subject it to whatever they recommend. It says that I do not know what to do for myself and that, no matter the financial cost or possible risk of further bodily harm, I trust them to do to my body whatever they see fit to figure it out. And they call my bluff every time, preemptively requiring me to sign a form legally releasing them of all liability, should anything they subject my body to result in further harm. This is literally a contract, giving their *business entity* the go-ahead to *experiment* on my body without responsibility for the outcome. It is a dangerous license to give any human, much less to a corporate entity, designed to protect the humans participating in it from liability. No one else truly knows *my body* and what it is experiencing better than *I myself*, the pilot of said body. My willingness to participate in this experimentation, by ingesting laboratory-derived drugs and approving *cutting-edge* treatments to be performed on my body, on the advice of a doctor alone, make it no wonder when compounding conditions result. I may one day come to a place with my body that this contract might make logical sense in my life, but until that day comes, I'd prefer not to take such a risk.

My body is solely my responsibility, and what I put in it or allow to have done to it is entirely my choice. If it is not actually broken, beyond its own ability to repair without assistance, then I am not going to try to have it fixed by relinquishing that control to anyone else, no matter their credentials. Taking my self-healing body to a doctor on a regular basis to see what they may find to fix—under the guise of *regular checkups*—makes about as much sense to me as going to a mechanic equally often and requesting they find something wrong with my smoothly running vehicle to charge me to repair. It is asking for unnecessary complications.

I no longer carry traditional health insurance because the frequency with which I am willing to attend makes it financially equivalent to only paying when something extreme enough happens to my body as to warrant my attendance. I also do not want to passively feed my income into a defunct system that then makes me feel that I have wasted my money if I do not attend. I don't believe that paying any amount of money into any system should bear any weight at all on whether I am inclined to seek medical assistance in the face of an injury or health condition, and the fact that I allowed it to do so for so much of my life is, to me, an indication of just how defunct this system is.

Understand I am *not* insinuating that we should abolish this system, as it has obviously resulted in some amazing discoveries and procedures, with regards to our bodies. What *I am* saying is that our attitude of perceived dependence on it, combined with the egotistical tendencies of the humans operating it, sets it up to create unnecessary health complications for us. We might all benefit from a revision of the foundational ideals upon which we have built this system.

Over the course of the eight months or so it has taken me to write this book, my body has been racked by countless pains, most of which I could see originated from some cut, abrasion, impact, or other damage I had inadvertently subjected it to, but a few of which I still cannot explain with any degree of certainty. One such pain occurred last November in my lower back region, mostly on the left side but a little bit on the right, as well. I first noticed it after a particularly strong workout, spurred by a spousal disagreement, so I thought maybe I had not been conscientious while doing side bends and had twisted slightly to the back, straining my lower back muscles. Over the following several nights, however, I found it painful enough to prevent me sleeping well. Upon waking one morning, Eleanor strongly suggested that I take myself in, fearing I may have a kidney infection. I decided to give it more time, of course—since that heals all wounds—and while I did, I remembered something that had happened to me a day or two prior to this pain registering.

It was a busy day, and while hustling on to my next errand, which involved the use of my truck bed, I discovered it full of kiteboarding gear from my previous adventure. Even one session involves a fair bit of gear since I have to go prepared with several kites for different possible wind conditions, so I had to carry a few armloads of stuff up the stairs and into a storage closet. This set me behind a few more minutes, so by the time I grabbed the last load of gear, which was all the way back in the far end of the bed, I was hurrying.

I drove a bigger Ford F-150 with a canopy topper and parked it in my steep driveway, facing uphill, so I had to climb up onto the tailgate and crawl to the back of the bed to fetch the gear, then drag it out with me and jump down. I thought, in my rush, that I might be just a tad bit faster if I clutched the bags close to me and then rolled back out, since it was downhill already, and I would not have to struggle so much. Unfortunately, I misjudged my momentum and rolled right off the end of the tailgate, falling three or four feet onto my back and landing mostly on my left side.

At the time, all I could do about it was pick myself up, have a good hearty laugh at my own expense, and carry on about my business, never once thinking back on it until this back pain several days later. Although it was entirely possible—even probable—that this had been the cause of the pain, it did not change my choice of what to do about it in the least. Whether it was this accident, improper workout technique, or the kidney infection Eleanor feared, time would heal all of them, so I did nothing, and within a few days it subsided and eventually disappeared altogether.

This brings me to my other mantra of good health: *ignore it and it will go away.*

Ignore It and It Will Go Away

This statement is not the call to carelessness that it suggests but rather an acknowledgment that our souls travel the universe in self-healing biological machines that quite efficiently repair themselves even as we carry on with our journey. Time ultimately heals all of our wounds, so once a wound has been determined not to require medical assistance (to heal more quickly or optimally), it need only be ignored and allowed to heal, without further damage.

Because we have so many signals informing us of pain or discomfort about which we may do nothing, the ability to ignore them is a necessity if we are to focus our conscious attention on the important tasks we still have to do despite them. Fretting over wounds that are already being repaired as best they can does not help them heal faster, but it does detract from our ability to *be here now.*

I first learned to *ignore it and it will go away* with my terrible facial acne as an early teen. It was fostered by a complete ignorance of personal hygiene—stemming from my hippie upbringing—and a tendency to pick profusely, gained from years of not being able to see clearly, beyond my face in the mirror. Not having cared for myself or what I looked like to others—nor having anyone else who cared, either—I struggled for years to have the self-control to stop myself from causing terrible damage to the skin of my face. At some point, I realized that every bit of it began just the same, with me walking by the mirror and deciding to stop and investigate that one big whitehead or that itchy rash spot I had been scratching. Once I leaned into the mirror, it all cascaded, leading me to a long string of subsequent pokings, pinchings, and proddings that would lead my body to have a whole lot more damage to repair than it ever had to begin with.

Once I had come to terms with this reality, there was only one way for me to overturn the bad habits of so many years, and it stared me blatantly in the face. I had to stop the first domino from ever falling, by not stopping at the mirror in the first place. So I planted a trigger by vividly imagining myself becoming aware that I was about to initiate the whole avalanche again the next time I walked by the mirror, but instead breaking the cycle by continuing to walk on by. I ignored the pains and discomforts of my facial acne until it so nearly went away that the only little zits remaining were irrelevant to me, since I never stopped to see them in the mirror anyway. It went amazingly far in improving my self-image, too, as I shed virtually all of my hyperactive teenage sense of self-consciousness in the process. I no longer give my body additional neurotic damage to heal from, and I have since adapted the technique to countless other aspects of my daily life. This might only have worked for me because my body did not begin growing facial hair in earnest until my mid-20s, otherwise I would have had to look at myself in the mirror daily to shave.

I ignore away a lifetime's infinity of minor injuries as they heal themselves and funnel any pains too strong to ignore into a more intense workout. This results in some overall muscle soreness, thereby masking the pain further and allowing me to continue eating up this life, voraciously. I am right now ignoring a pulled Achilles tendon in my left heel, an inflammation in my right middle

141

finger (middle knuckle), a minor displacement of my right hip, a chronically bruised left funny bone—from always knocking it on door jambs—and my jaw is sprained on the left from biting confidently into a smoked turkey leg that was not nearly so tender as I had presumed. This is in addition to all of the normal aches and pains of having a 40-year-old body I have continually put through the wringer like there is no tomorrow.

I also ignore away a majority of illnesses I acquire, from seasonal coughs and colds to food poisoning and stomach bugs not severe enough to cause vomiting or diarrhea. I try not to even concede to myself that I am feeling unwell until I know I am beyond the climax of it, so I have only to coast into the nearby light at the end of my tunnel. If I am worried my body is feeling unwell enough for me to not be able to work out in the days that follow, then I work out especially hard one day after the next, sometimes right up until I have pushed my body all the way through it. I dislike feeling weak, so when days come in which I *am* too sick to work out, the moment I feel able to work out again, I do, so as to minimize the atrophy my body experiences and invigorate my immune response. I greatly appreciate coming to the end of an illness to find my body stronger for having had it. Every challenge in this life is an opportunity to shine.

Since powering my way through most health adversity is a given for me, feeling strong is far more important than actually being strong, particularly when it comes to illness. A firm belief I am feeling strong leads me to have a vigorous activity level, which in turn distracts me from my pains and discomforts, while bolstering my body's ability to heal from whatever is ailing it. The moment I have accepted that I am, in fact, feeling unwell is the beginning of a downward trend in my activity level that results in a cascade of negative physiological fallout, including a compromised immune response and the muscular atrophy of lying in bed feeling pathetic. No one likes that, so I find ways to consciously distract myself from such things until they are forgotten, effectively going away.

Physical, real-world tasks are the best distraction tools I have found for ignoring pain or infirmity because giving my brain a task that consumes most of its desktop memory prevents it from having the attention left to dwell too intently on the pain messages it is receiving. This is why, when I begin to think my body may be coming down with an illness or I have just injured it harshly in a way that does not require assistance, I promptly find myself an all-consuming task to delve deeply into. Because this technique is all about distracting the brain from its many signal inputs, the more of my senses (sight, sound, smell, touch, and so on) that are engaged by my choice of tasks, the more effective it is at masking the perception of pain.

I have seen other humans use breathing toward the same end. During some of the more painful medical procedures I have endured, medical professionals have coached me to focus intently on my breathing as a means of distracting myself from the pain. This serves to ensure that my brain has enough oxygen, to prevent me passing out, and also to increase both respiration and circulation, allowing for maximum cleansing of the waste metabolites associated with repair. My yoga instructor in college also encouraged breathing as an effective distraction from the pain of particularly intense stretches, and I have seen birthing mothers coached in the same way.

Of course, attempting to *ignore it and it will go away* with every injury and sickness eventually gets me into trouble, which is why listening to my body is so important: to hear when it is telling me that it *actually* needs assistance.

When You've Gotta Go, You've Gotta Go

There have been a few times in my adult life when I have been unable to avoid receiving medical assistance for my body, and they were all serious. Looking back, however, I am not entirely certain that they all truly warranted the trip.

When we first moved to Oregon 13 years ago, I got the job working grave-yard shift at a local mill, making plywood on the assembly line. I was about eight months into the job and had just come to terms with the harsh reality that I would not see healthy sleep again, until I found other employment. Unfortunately, we were several months away from moving to a bigger city where other employment opportunities might be found, leaving me to power through it as best I could to support myself and my family.

The shift started at 11 p.m., but I usually got out of bed about eight o'clock since the mill was 25 minutes away. I would have coffee and pack myself a lunch, nibble on some dinner leftovers for "breakfast," and head out the door, not to return until eight the next morning.

This being my first winter in a temperate climate in more than a decade, after my stints in Hawaii and Florida, working through the nights in an open-air hangar during the cold winter nights compromised my immune system. I had been unable to shake off my most recent cough for weeks, and it had come after a long string of other minor illnesses that had begun in the fall.

One night, Eleanor came in to kiss me awake and tell me it was time to get up for work, but, despite my feeling just fine in the moment, when I swung my feet out of bed onto the floor, my knees buckled under me and I fell, feeling suddenly weak and dizzy. She tried to help me up, but I declined, insisting I was alright. I attempted several times to make my body get up and carry me into the shower, but every time my head came off the floor I became dizzy, and attempting to get on my feet made the world sway back and forth like a rocking ship until I fell over again. Eleanor supported me with her shoulder, helping to walk me the few steps into the bathroom, but by the time we got there my body had gone limp. She oozed me off of her and into the bathtub, drawing me a bath while she called the local urgent care clinic.

They advised her to bring me in, so she hung up the phone and called my foreman at work. When she put the cellphone to my ear for me to express to him my situation, I could barely utter single-syllable words and struggled to make them loud enough for him to perceive over the loud din of machinery I knew he had in the background. After the bath, I felt a little better but still had to lie down in bed awhile before I could be convinced to journey downstairs and outside to the minivan.

At the urgent care clinic, they did some tests and concluded that I had walking pneumonia and had been working in the cold, with a low-grade fever, for who knows how long. I was prescribed antibiotics and a few days off work, which seemed to do the trick, but I did not feel my immunity bounce fully back until I was able to get us moved to the bigger city of Beaverton months later—and back on a waiter's sleep schedule.

I do not like taking antibiotics for the same reason I do not like using hand sanitizer. The healthy balance of our bodies is maintained, in part, by a symbiotic relationship with the microbial populations they sustain, and both antibiotics and hand sanitizer utterly destroy those populations in the microbiomes they inhabit (our guts and our skin, respectively). Not to mention, the naturalist in me knows that if it does not exist in nature, our bodies do not *need* it, so using these products on our bodies may well result in them having to do more work than they otherwise would to reestablish balance. I have taken antibiotics only a handful of times in my life, and most of those were when I was a kid.

Taking personal responsibility for what I allow into my body requires an acknowledgment that *I alone* am the first, last, and only decision-maker when it comes to the ingestion of anything—whether medicinal, nourishing, or otherwise. This is why I am prone to neurotically inspect every glass, dish, and piece of silverware before I use it, as I am ever-conscious that once I have put it into my mouth, I have no one to blame but myself for what may have been on it.

Right around age 30, my body began telling me that what Eleanor had spent years telling me already was, unfortunately, true: our bodies eventually get older and less elastic, regardless of how strongly we try to believe our way around it. During this time, my body pushed out a hernia, acquired an aversion to spicy peppers and caffeine, and also made me painfully aware of a new threshold in its tolerance to stress.

One summer afternoon, just after working out, Eleanor and I went to take a walk together in the sunshine, and I felt my abdomen feeling kind of loose and uncomfortable. When I stripped down to shower on arrival back home, I discovered a huge new lump in my lower abdominal, upper groin area on the left side. Needless to say, I was a bit freaked out, but that alone was not enough to spur me into a doctor visit.

I diagnosed myself with an inguinal hernia all of half an hour later, after a quick internet search. This is basically a tear in the abdominal membrane—usually due to the intense abdominal pressure of coughing, sneezing, or lifting something heavy—into which organs or other tissues are subsequently pushed, leading to a notable protrusion. I promptly stopped working out and spent the next couple of weeks combing through accounts, both in person and online, and picking the brains of everyone I could find who had experience with a hernia.

I discovered that men and women both get them, but men are much more prone to them due to the particulars of our internal development. About 25 percent of men will have one in their lives (only 3 percent of women), and before surgical methods were determined to patch them, they were a common cause of death. Even today, many people die from them or from complications arising from them. During my research, I learned that my boss at work had been avoiding surgery for a hernia for over five years. I also met someone whose friend had put it off for over 30 years, after which time major surgery was necessary to correct the extensive internal and external damage it had caused. I decided medical intervention was necessary if I was to continue living a fulfilling life, for myself and my young family.

By the time I got the surgery scheduled, six months had passed, making this the longest break my body has ever had from working out in its entire adult existence. The surgeon I was assigned to through insurance adopted a now-familiar attitude with me, being downright condescending in his certainty that my lack of medical credentials meant I could not possibly know what was *actually happening* with my own body. He required only a five-minute assessment to confirm my diagnosis.

The day of the surgery was all very hazy and surreal for me, but I distinctly remember how it all went down once I was admitted. Eleanor drove me to the surgery center, of course, since I was to be put under and the anesthetic was expected to wear off over the course of the rest of the day. I was promptly asked to dress down, put on a hospital gown, and lie in a bed to have an IV put in, after which my surgeon came in to go over with us what would happen.

As he wrapped up, the anesthesiologist came in and released the anesthetic into my IV. I began to get groggy as the surgeon took out a red marker and drew a big "X" on my lower abdomen, but when you have a hernia and you lie on your back, gravity pulls everything back in so it does not show. I was too out of it to notice or be capable of speaking, but as my consciousness drifted out, I heard Eleanor next to me—as if from far, far away—say to the surgeon in a blood-curdling tone, "You know it's on the other side, right?! I *love* this man. If you f*@# him up, I *will* be waiting for you in the parking lot when you get off work . . ."

Even long after recovery, I still only rarely indulge in leg-lifts because I feel them tease up the edges of my internal mesh patch and also because I feel the propensity for a hernia to pop out on the other side of my abdomen, with the particular strain they cause. My tummy is no longer as trim as it was in my youth, but this does not affect my strength or flexibility in daily activity.

My other 30-year reality check came in the spring, during finals week of my last term in community college, before I was to transfer up to Portland State University in the fall. Eleanor had just asked me to help her build a neighborhood coffee shop out of a one-bedroom apartment in downtown Beaverton while we juggled our now eight- and nine-year-old boys and I worked a full-time server position in a downtown Portland restaurant.

I have always had a meticulous tendency, which served me well in school and in my service career, but which made the unending tide of mess in a home life dominated by two high-energy young boys uniquely stressful for me, as I was forever trying to beat back this tide.

As I undertook more and more responsibility, my tendency to push harder, taking every challenge as an opportunity to overcome, continued to increase my body's stress response. From my perspective, I was young, I was strong, and there was no good reason why I could not take on and efficiently handle everything life could throw at me. I did not have as much time for sleep as my body prefers, and I drank a lot of caffeine to remain alert through many consecutive long days with many stressors, while wearing many different hats.

My meticulousness blazed fiercely through my studies, so I had managed to maintain a perfect grade point average throughout my entire college career, even with my life's other constraints. I flipped methodically through my biology flashcards while fighting morning traffic on the way to take the final, when I was suddenly gripped by a building sense of panic. As it grew, I became aware of an internal pain growing with it, somewhere in the vicinity of my butt. I broke out in a profuse cold sweat and could no longer tolerate the pain of sitting directly on my bottom, instead pushing frantically at the seat beneath me to relieve the pressure, while maintaining control of the minivan. At stop lights, I used both hands to lift myself off the seat and gain the relief I had to have if I was to continue the battle for the remainder of the drive. This continued for the last five minutes of my morning commute but felt like an absolute eternity.

Parking on campus was one place I could squeeze a bit of overhead out of my tight, parental student budget, so my practice was to park several blocks away and walk in, adding more pressure to an already intense situation. On this day, I sat in the car just long enough to compose myself before attempting the walk but was still unable to make it even the first two blocks. A woman I saw regularly, who lived in one of the houses I walked past, came out with her fluffy white Pomeranian on a red leash, bound for a walk of their own. After locking her front door, she turned to face the street and discovered me doubled over and crouched down on the side of the road—flashcards in hand—moaning in pain.

"Oh no, what's the matter?" she asked me with sincere concern.

"I'm fine," I replied through tight lips. "I just need to get to my final."

"No, no, sweetie," she replied in a nurturing, motherly tone, "you just need to turn yourself around right now and take yourself back home. Do you need some help to get back to your car?" I declined and spent the next ten minutes working my way slowly back to the minivan, between bouts of crippling pain. By the time I finally returned home to our third-floor walkup apartment, the pain was so bad I literally crawled up the last flight of stairs, drawing the attention of a neighbor, who helped me through it. A few moments later, Eleanor helped me back down the stairs after calling ahead to the local urgent care clinic. It was to be the last time I left the apartment for more than two weeks.

At the clinic, I received a prostate exam from a bashful, attractive young female doctor, while my wife stood next to me for emotional support. After a brief exam, the doctor hurriedly pronounced it an enlarged prostate and left the room awkwardly, informing me as she went of a CT scan and some other tests she would like to have run to confirm the diagnosis. I allowed them to conduct their tests and went home, where I spent much of the next several days soaking in a hot bath.

After three days, I was still in too much pain to walk and had not heard from the urgent care clinic to confirm their doctor's diagnosis and give me some guidance toward a return to normalcy. I called, and the receptionist said he would pass my message on to the doctor. When I did not hear back by the following afternoon, I called again, explaining my situation to the receptionist. He asked me to hold while he went to speak with the doctor about it, returning a few minutes later to say that all tests had come out fine and there was nothing wrong with me.

"That's great," I said. "So why am I still in so much pain then?!" He put me on hold to go speak with the doctor once again and returned to give me the only clue my $5,000 worth of testing got me: "She says, look up *levator syndrome*." I did, and discovered something interesting about my body. While most people's bodies tend to hold their stress in the neck and shoulders, the space between the eyebrows, or another common place, my body instead holds its stress in the pelvic floor muscle. This is a hammock-shaped muscle residing within the pelvis, which cradles the prostate and bladder, among other innards.

Levator syndrome is historically a perfectionist young man's disorder, in which the stress of not being able to make things *just so* leads to incrementally more and more severe subconscious tensing of the pelvic floor muscle. My body's particularly nasty response to this condition was exacerbated by my continually increasing stress load, coupled with deep-tissue dehydration from too much caffeine throughout the day and alcohol to unwind at night, without enough water in between. Cramping of my pelvic floor muscle escalated to a cascade of rolling cramps running through my digestive tract, which rendered me incapable of doing anything but lying in a hot bath day after day, for weeks.

Over the course of these weeks—after quitting all caffeine and alcohol, eating only room-temperature food, including a hefty increase of plant matter, and learning to be in touch with the musculature of my innards through meditation—my condition finally eased up enough for me to return to functionality. Of course, my straight-A GPA dropped to Bs and Cs across the board, and my perfect attendance record at school and work were tragically tarnished as well.

For the last ten years, I have yo-yoed between periods of living this bland, unstressed, caffeine- and alcohol-free life—for the sake of inner recuperation—interspersed with periods through which I feel good enough to gradually increase these factors to a point of near-normalcy, before being painfully reminded again that my body is not like everyone else's. Now, my body has *also* developed a prematurely enlarged prostate for me to juggle, forcing me to adapt by omitting coffee altogether and drinking ceremonial-grade matcha green tea in the mornings instead. I still yo-yo with alcohol, but I feel my body telling me that its days, too, are numbered.

Resuming a normal life after the jarring experience of coming to terms with my stress disorder also required that I come to terms with the truth about perfection. Perfection is a construct of the human mind and is entirely relative to the eyes of the beholder, similar to beauty. Even the definition—the state, condition, or quality of being as free as possible from all flaws or defects—acknowledges that, like facts and truth, perfection is relative to what is possible at the time the thing being described as such exists. Different humans will know this thing more or less intimately, leading to different opinions of what it may be perfect for. If there's anything I know as a human, it's that there is always room for improvement, even if it means constantly chasing innovation. In the physical, anything we might choose to term as perfect may be dissected into the smaller and smaller nested building blocks of matter making it up, until it reaches a point we would deem grossly imperfect. When viewed through an electron microscope, even the cleanest of lines is just a frayed mess of atomic particles, loosely organizing themselves into a dynamic array that is constantly shifting in response to the constantly shifting particles surrounding them.

Everything in this universe is truly relative to *everything else* in this universe, and it is our particular and ever-changing mental and physical perspectives that allow us to perceive the objects and experiences of our lives as we do. Expecting perfection anywhere in our universe is a human paradox we have set up for ourselves, like so many others. I am now forced to express my meticulousness with a less-insistent edge that acknowledges perfection as the unattainable asymptote that it is, for the sake of my health.

CHAPTER 7
Recovery Options

When we are done being sick, injured, or having surgery, a period of recovery is normal for the body to regain its previous vigor. In the case of sickness, this involves a return to normal diet and the gradual return to a healthy weight, including the rebuilding of atrophied muscles. It also includes the body healing itself from whatever side effects were produced by the illness, like bedsores or a scratchy throat. With injuries or surgery, this usually includes behavioral adjustments intended to avoid the risk of reinjury, like changing techniques for lifting or even eliminating particular activities altogether. Behavioral adaptations of this nature are open-ended, so they may return to normal gradually over a long time, suddenly over a short time, or never.

No matter the ailment, choices must be made with regard to recovery. Resting allows the body to use the energy it would otherwise spend being productive to heal itself more quickly instead. Unfortunately, the more resting a body does, the more it becomes unaccustomed to the average stresses of a normal activity level, therefore making it a more uphill climb to regain its original degree of vigor. I do whatever I feel capable of doing, even as I recover from my multitude of infirmities, because it means more of my time is spent living a full life, and my body does eventually make a complete recovery regardless. I am aware that I choose this at the expense of an optimally expedient recovery, but I don't like feeling weak or incapable, which increases incrementally as I diminish my activity level to accommodate any injury or sickness.

I remember going in for a follow-up appointment two weeks after my hernia surgery, when I was no longer inclined to continue lying around, despite Eleanor and my boss collaborating to prevent me returning to work for another week yet. I entered the doctor's office explaining right off that I was used to a lot of activity and had stopped doing anything strenuous months ago over this, so if he would not mind terribly just writing me up a permission slip so I could go on about my business killing it . . . please. After an inspection of the surgery site, he proudly proclaimed me free to do just that.

"Really?!" I exclaimed in disbelief. "Because if you're *serious*, I'm working out as soon as I get home!"

He nodded in approval.

"And I'm biking the 12 miles to work again, starting tomorrow!" I said excitedly, feeling out just how far I could go.

Again he gave his seal of approval, saying in response, "Give it your worst. I am confident it will hold."

I made him put it in writing and carried it with me for the next week, to present to anyone who tried to insist I should not be pushing so hard.

There are choices to be made with regard to medication as well, no matter the condition. The simplest choice is of course not to medicate at all, which has a high probability of working out just fine, thanks to our elegantly efficient, self-healing bodies. If an ailment does not recover without medication, then chances are good the body is deficient in something essential, like a particular mineral, contact with the planet, or enough sleep or water. Stress responses are widely varied and may be quite extreme, providing explanation for most of the other mysterious responses of the body.

The most obvious medication choice is to accept and ingest whatever prescription drug a doctor recommends and prescribes for a particular condition, but in many cases, they are being given financial incentives to do so by the drug companies providing them. I know this because I have served many pharmaceutical-funded dinner parties, clearly intended to coerce the doctors invited—through nice steaks, lobster tails, and expensive wines—to prescribe their drugs. At these events, I have even witnessed offers of direct financial compensation per patient. Even when this is not the case, the drug companies themselves are in constant competition with one another to conceive of the next best medication to treat a given issue, each iteration of which comes complete with its own list of side effects, some of which—they are willing to openly admit—might just kill some of us. These side effects are good for the medical industry because they give us more issues for them to treat with more medications, which they have definitely conceived of already. This illustrates the obvious downfall of just taking whatever you are prescribed: it may lead you to be caught up in this cycle indefinitely, or at least until you feel able to quit them all, cold turkey.

The more natural option for medication is the nearly infinite supply of healing plants and fungi our world provides, most of which have co-evolved with us to provide our bodies with well-rounded nourishment and a hearty immune system. Many of today's pharmaceutical drugs are purified compounds, derived directly from these plants and fungi, inducing more severe side effects only because they have been taken out of their context and concentrated far beyond their natural occurrence. Just as the robustness of our bodies is dependent on their constant interaction with the intricate web of other critters amongst which they have arisen, the curative molecules in plants and fungi are most balanced and potent for our bodies when they are combined with the many other interactive substances with which they naturally occur. Teasing them out of the organisms that produce them to purify and create pills out of them—in highly unnatural concentrations—may well produce powerful results within our systems, but it does not surprise me in the least that some of those effects are also highly undesirable. This is why I revert to trailside foraging for the vegetative complement of my diet at times when my body is experiencing unusual symptoms for which I cannot readily find a solution.

I recently spent a couple of months figuring out the solution to managing my prematurely enlarged prostate, beyond the behavioral adaptation of emptying it more often to relieve the pressure. I first did some research to find out the many possible natural treatments for my condition, like ashwagandha, pumpkin seeds, stinging nettle, krill oil, the red-belted conk fungus, reishi, saw palmetto, and pygeum bark. I found wild local sources to personally forage as many as possible and began testing their effects on my symptoms, one by one. When none of them solved my problems, I then began the same trial-and-error process with the ones available as unpurified supplements—like saw palmetto leaves and ashwagandha root—sold as actual dried plant material put into capsules.

During this time, I began most days with a hike up into the woods with my dogs to graze on my favorite trailside plants, as shifting the diet to more vege-tative matter and less meat has been shown to help some men suffering from this condition. I also did this because all of the plants available in the grocery stores have been genetically modified—if only through selective breeding over many generations—to select for traits like larger size, insect resistance, and faster development times. They no longer contain quite the same combinations or proportions of substances that they originally did in the wild. Since my body is designed to consume the naturally occurring plant matter of our planet, the more I ingest modified organisms instead, the further away it gets from its natural balance. Not so much as ingesting only Pepsi and cigarette smoke, of course, but certainly enough to produce subtle signs of internal imbalance, like a prostate that becomes chronically enlarged about a decade earlier than is statistically expected.

Since I am not a primitive human, I also spent this time exploring other naturally occurring treatments from other places in the world, which is how I finally discovered the ceremonial-grade matcha green tea that now allows me to manage my prostate in the way I prefer. Being a modern human with a natu-ralist perspective, I am constantly considering and reconsidering how best to ride the fine line between maintaining my human body in the most naturally healthy state possible and enjoying the most fulfilling modern human experi-ence I can. Before I resume this discourse on recovery options, I would like to delve a bit deeper into the topic of foraging wild vegetation.

When foraging, I browse from only the most vigorous individual plants and only from their most healthy-looking foliage. This is because they are more likely to contain a higher concentration of well-made components and also because selecting only the healthiest ingredients from which to build and maintain my body is a reflection of my actual care for self. I also do not rinse them but rather select leaves from higher up where less dirt and dust has accrued on them, and I blow or wipe off any dirt I do see on them with my fingers before consuming them. I do this because the naturalist in me knows that our primitive ancestors—who were healthy enough to spawn modern man—did not have the microbial awareness to rinse from their food the healthy balance of naturally occurring microbes found both on its surface and in the microscopic bits of soil stuck to it. Consciously ingesting these microbes helps keep my system hearty and well-practiced in contending with the full spectrum of life with which it is intended to interact. This is in contrast to my microbial behavior in the human world, because there, the probability of a given microbe being pathogenic to my particular body is so much higher.

By my estimation of it—after a lifetime of wild foraging—around 60 percent of the tender flora in our environment is edible for our bodies, with a bit of variation depending on the given ecosystem type (desert, forest, rainforest, and so on) and season. In fact, as with spicy peppers, our bodies are capable of building a tolerance to many plants that have evolved substances within them intended to deter us from consuming them. Our bodies can even build a tolerance to plants that we consider overtly toxic, given enough dilution in a wide variety of other foods. So much edible plant life exists all around us that being a good forager is more about being comfortable trying things and learning what *not* to eat—or how plants must be prepared before eating them—than it is about learning all of the ones you *can* eat. I learned to forage plants for myself at a very young age, mostly from naturally inclined trial and error. I'm even told that when I was two, my family once watched me casually pick up and eat a large banana slug.

Trying foraged foods is not as casual as it sounds but rather involves gradually introducing them to the body by first crushing and rubbing them lightly on the lips, then waiting several minutes to observe any reaction before moistening the lips and doing it again. If it passes these tests with no adverse effects—like stinging, burning, or rash—then it graduates to a test on the tongue and then to chewing and spitting out a bit. Finally comes ingestion, incrementally and with time to observe the system's response between each increment. Nearly everything may be toxic in enough quantity (or concentration), so moderation and variation are the general rule of thumb. *Every body* responds differently to *every thing*, and food preferences, aversions, intolerances and allergies are normal responses, whether they be to wild foraged or processed foods. I apply this testing process to all foods that I forage, even ones that are commonly known to be edible among the masses. A vegetarian diet is akin to a default setting for the body of a hunter-gatherer that is unmotivated or otherwise unsuccessful at hunting, so keeping up with my foraging abilities ensures that whatever happens in the human hive, I always have the choice to walk away, should I decide I want to.

Returning now to the subject of recovery, beyond medication options, recovery also requires choices be made with regard to activity. This includes both the rate at which activity level is returned to normal and behavioral modifications to prevent reinjury or resurgence of sickness. If possible, I try my best not to reduce my activity level to begin with so my body's internal balance is least thrown off in the first place, and therefore the least possible amount of chemical work is required for it to reestablish its balance. If I am forced to reduce activity level, then I simply do my best to minimize that reduction and begin the process of returning it to its start point as soon as it is feasible to do so. This means I sometimes find myself systematically flexing and relaxing each muscle group while I lie in bed recovering from sickness or injury, awaiting the full return of my body's energy as I also build it up through use.

I apply behavioral modifications after an injury or sickness on a case-by-case basis. My shoulders are a good example of this because I have separated both of them multiple times, so my workout routine has been modified for their sake just as many times.

The first separation happened to my left shoulder while snowboarding as a teenager, somewhere around 16 or so. It was not too bad—grade 1, by medical terminology—and I was young, strong, and resilient, so I just skipped push-ups, chest presses, and tricep dips for a week and a half or so while I kept it in a sling. At the time, I was a dishwasher at a local brewpub, so I had to modify my technique for moving tall, heavy stacks of plates and glass racks, using mostly my right arm to cradle them and my injured left one to keep them balanced. I made a full recovery within a month, and so did my workout routine and my work techniques.

Then, when I was about 25 and we were living in Sarasota, Florida, I had a high-speed collision on my bicycle with a stop light post to avoid a careless driver, while hustling to work. Because I saw it coming, I slid to the side to buffer myself, taking the brunt of the impact against my right shoulder, which sustained a grade 2 separation. This one was a little more serious, and I was not quite so young and elastic, so I did skip a few days of work, and although I mostly recovered within a month or so, full recovery happened slowly, over the course of the next couple of years. I leaned heavily on my bussers at work for a few months, tipping them out a bit extra to keep them aggressive about plate-clearing in my section, so as not to compromise my shoulder with stacks of heavy plateware.

Rehabilitation required adjustments to my workout routine that I have continued ever since, including both fore and lateral arm raises and my swim-stroke-emulating rotator cuff exercise. These were necessary to bring my shoulder back up to full functionality, but I have retained them because I can feel that doing them maintains my shoulders in a more stout condition overall, thereby diminishing the probability I may injure them again.

After my worst shoulder injury—a grade 4 separation, from the skateboarding accident just a few years back—I adjusted my workout routine again. This time, I added what is known as an eccentric shoulder external rotation. I had to stop doing tricep dips as well, and for six months or so, even push-ups and chest presses were out. As an additional behavioral modification, I have now trained my body to reflexively clench my shoulders in anticipation of possible impending tugs or jerks—much like instinctively holding my breath before my head plunges under the water during kiteboarding wipeouts. I also avoid any skateboard that is not a longboard, and I no longer mountain bike, to avoid jamming my shoulders in a short-stop or collision scenario. Truly, I could still do these activities, but I am starkly conscious that doing so would put at risk my future years of kiteboarding, and that's not worth it to me.

My weakest side—which sets the pace in workouts—flip-flopped back and forth throughout these years of injury, in terms of my upper body. My left shoulder still has subtle weakness in particular ways, as it hangs off me like a sagging, tweaked gate hinge.

Many of my personal health philosophies have drawn negative criticism from my loved ones, who fear I am doing myself more harm than good and perhaps even leading my body to a premature demise. In response, I have voiced to them my concerns that they may be doing themselves more harm than good in holding back—attempting to preserve a physical self that may well be destined for its own premature demise—thereby forgoing the potential richness of their lives for fear of taking damage. Our bodies are all predestined to age, degrade, and die, regardless of how much we are or are not able to preserve them from damage. For this reason, I ask those concerned with my beliefs to consider the real-life evidence of human health histories like that of Evel Knievel, for whom the Guinness World Record keepers created the new category of "most broken bones in a lifetime," or Jack LaLanne, who at age 70 personally tugged 70 rowboats a mile across Long Beach Harbor, one of them with several passengers aboard. Their personal health philosophies led them to intensely rich lives, filled with overwhelming physical accomplishments and equally overwhelming bodily damage, yet both still died old men, of natural causes.

TAKEAWAY MESSAGES

So, what's my secret? How do I find myself to be living so casually in this buff, 40-year-old, highly functional but largely broken human body while paying little notable attention to my health?

My lifetime has taught me that the care and maintenance of my human body's health is instinctively built into me and is innately simple but has required that I learn to listen to what it is telling me and then learn to filter and prioritize its messages.

I consider what is natural for my body and provide it with a diversity of appropriate nourishment. I also consider what is natural for my soul and provide it with appropriate nourishment as well. If my body behaves anomalously, I check in first with its basic needs, then check in with the other humans around me and see what may or may not have worked for them under similar circumstances. Same with my spirit.

I maintain my optimal physical self in all regards, so the only thing limiting me is my own will. I live my life with the reckless abandon of a being contained within a self-healing biological machine because that is what I am.

My mother's early demise has served as a constant reminder throughout my life that our lives here are not guaranteed for any particular period of time. This has led me to an understanding that every moment I find myself having is precious enough to make the most of. I try to keep myself in perspective with regard to the life around me and to be conscious of as much as possible, all the time.

I am mindful of the foods and liquids I ingest for my body's growth and maintenance, not just to avoid ingesting something unhealthy for me but also because paying attention to it helps my body to better process and utilize it. I am present as I go about my daily activities both to avoid missteps and also to ensure that I have a more complete awareness of the infinite opportunities constantly flowing by. I do my best to *be here now* because anything I do in my present with the subconscious distractions of my future or my past running through my head results in that thing being done with less efficiency; that is, I cannot be doing my true best. If I feel the need to reflect upon my past or to plan for my future, I make time to think consciously about it, so even *this* may receive my complete and present-minded attention, to be all that it may. This applies to everything.

I sincerely strive to appreciate every present moment as deeply as possible, embracing the downfalls of my life for the growth opportunities they provide as much as I do the climaxes for all of their glory. I recognize that I will probably come to look back at this moment from many random moments in the future, some of which are bound to be better and others of which are certain to be worse.

I am honest and true to myself so the efforts of my life may be succinct and so that my self-respect may amplify those efforts. If I don't like something about myself, I change it, since I'm the only one who can.

I believe myself strong without hesitation, in both spirit and body, and let my actions support that belief. I build up and exercise my sense of *I can* to stave off all of those pesky, excuse-driven *I can'ts*. *Believing* I am strong is more important than actually *being* strong because I can be as physically strong as I want to be, but if I believe I am weak, then my actions will reaffirm this belief. This is the power of the psychosomatic response. Since my body responds so strongly to my expectations of it, believing I feel vigorous and healthy also leads it to express just that. Stressing about my health is, therefore, counterproductive to being in good health.

I hope to believe myself strong and healthy until the moment I die, so my life may be marked by the least possible amount of weakness and self-doubt. Should my body fall prey to the cancer of my family's genetic proclivity, my only hope would be that I be too busy living an active and fulfilled life to notice it in the least. Because we know that it may one day come to pass, it has—by necessity—crossed the family discussion table several times, and my wife and children are clear where I stand on the issue. Maybe my body is riddled with cancer right this moment, but if I feel happy, healthy, and well-adjusted from now until the day I die, what does it really matter?

I will not choose to die the slow and painful death of my mother, allowing my loved ones to remember me as a suffering shell of a person, clinging to whatever hope the medical industry could offer me, all the way to the bitter end. If my diagnosis should come, I will immediately drop everything to prepare for my trek—by bare feet—to the Amazon Rainforest, so my soul may enjoy the satisfaction of what could be my final adventure to my ultimate bucket-list destination. I will plot a course through the wilderness, avoiding roads and civilization, to whatever extent is possible. Along the way, my body will experience a complete immersion in its naturally intended environment, satisfying its instinctive drive to hunt, gather, and navigate the wilds while enjoying the holistically natural and balanced diet that results. It will inhale only fresh, outside air and feel the energy of the sun, both on its skin and through the replenishing flow of free electrons its rays excite from the Earth.

Through this cleansing process, I would hope to reset my physiology, thereby supporting my body to make every best attempt at solving its own problem, naturally. Should I arrive at my destination healthy and strong, I will presume my body to have beaten its adversary and begin a new chapter of my life, and if I do not, then I will have enjoyed the intensity of the journey—all the way to the finish line.

Being the kind of human who would rather burn out than fade away, this contingency plan is more of a worst-case scenario, as my optimal death would be something truly thrilling, like riding a wingsuit headlong into a big tornado. My family knows I do not wish to die an invalid, whether hooked up to a life-support system in a hospital bed or expiring passively in an elder-care facility. They know that, in either of these cases, I will need them to sneak in a rip-snorting mean grizzly bear to give me the exhilarating death of a lifetime, or rustle up something else along those lines. However, in the meantime, so long as I still only have a limited time to live and I do not get to know when my time is up, I intend to continue living out my life to the absolute fullest.

Since all of life could be seen as a never-ending series of problems to be solved, this means getting good at problem-solving and learning to manage my expectations. In other words, *hoping* for the best but *expecting* the worst, and with a conscious eye to the fact that, as bad as anything is, it can always get worse—right up until the moment I am not here anymore.

It also means awakening my instincts and continuing to listen avidly to them, since my spirit is the only pilot of my body, and no one else on the planet can ever know either one as well as I do. Listening to my instincts is the best way for me to care for the body I have been born into and to lead myself to greater spiritual fulfillment.

When I step into the wilds and am enveloped by our bodies' naturally intended environment, it becomes clear to me that our modern urban landscape provides our human organism with an excess of stimulation, overwhelming our brains and resulting in neurotic stress disorders, systemwide. I frequently take the time to step into the wilderness, take off my socks and shoes, and plug myself in to nature's web, to awaken the instincts of my body and my soul and then to consider, without fear, whatever actions they may drive me to.

I have learned myself and figured out what thrills me enough to give my life meaning, then given it everything I've got, and when it has changed, I have changed with it. I have let this be what leads my life. I engage my universe by keeping an open mind, paying conscious attention to my life's road signs, and being brave enough to follow them. I refuse to disengage my universe until my time is up.

When I consider what I would like for readers of this book to come away with, a few predominant ideas come to mind. Treat life with a care that demonstrates an awareness of its value, be it your own or that of another. Be ever conscious and thankful—not careless—for the life we all get to share with one another in these moments of history to which we make our individual contributions. As omnivorous animals, we can't exist without literally consuming certain other organisms, but the degree to which each of us affect the lives of the remaining creatures of this Earth plays out in our individual choices, moment to moment.

You do not have to look so far as the few remaining indigenous tribal cultures of the world to find perfectly healthy people who have never before seen a doctor. Multitudes of them live in deep-country areas all over the world, and many of them live long and excessively productive lives. Generally speaking, our bodies do not *need* perpetual medical treatment, and how much they *do* need is determined by our perception and beliefs about it. Do your best to satisfy your body's needs, think positively, and learn to manage its many stress responses so you do not create issues where there otherwise are none.

Our perception determines our reality, and we choose, to a large extent, what we believe we have perceived. Whether we choose to perceive a positive world around us or a negative one, our bodies reinforce those perceptions through hormones and the adjustment of physiologic momentum. This means that much of how we feel is within our own control.

Nowhere in its inception did the give-and-take concept of treating others as you would have them treat you ever say anything about it being an exclusively human-applying principle. Have compassion for the ails of your own human condition when you see them in those around you, but also try to have compassion for the ails of your animal—and even your basic organismal—conditions as well. *All* life is precious and deserves to be treated as such.

Like the ideas in this book, nothing in this life is set in stone; rather, change is the only thing that is certain and constant. Consider every occurrence of your life with an open mind and on a case-by-case basis, because being set in your ways prevents you from flowing freely with your universe.

Be a conscious pilot of your body, and keep things in perspective. Choose to think of *how* you can instead of *why* you can't and truly do your best, because in a life where every breath you take and every opportunity you're offered could literally be your last, there is no *good* reason why you *can't*. After all, life is out there to be lived, so discover yourself, find your strength, get out there and live it with everything you've got!

GLOSSARY

Accrue *v.* be received in regular or increasing amounts

Accumulate *v.* gather together a number or quantity; increase

Acuity *n.* sharpness of thought, vision, or hearing

Acutely *adv.* sharply; keenly

Adapt *v.* make something suitable for a new purpose; become adjusted to new conditions

Adequately *adv.* satisfactorily or acceptably; sufficiently

ADHD *abbr.* attention deficit hyperactivity disorder

Adrenaline *n.* hormone produced by the adrenal glands in response to stress that makes the body's natural processes work more quickly

Advent *n.* the arrival of an important person or thing

Adverse *adj.* harmful or unfavorable

Adversity *n.* a difficult or unpleasant situation; misfortune

Aloe vera *n.* a jellylike substance obtained from a type of Aloe, used to soothe the skin

Aloft *adv.* up in or into the air; overhead

Amino acid *n.* any of the natural substances that combine to form proteins

Amplify *v.* increase the strength of

Anecdotes *n.* a short entertaining story about a real incident or person

Anesthesiologist *n.* a doctor who specializes in administering a drug or gas that makes you unable to feel pain

Anesthetic *n.* a drug or gas that makes you unable to feel pain

Anomalous *adj.* differing from what is standard or normal

Anterior *adj.* at or near the front

Anticipate *v.* be aware of and prepared for a future event

Apathetic *adj.* not interested or enthusiastic

Apathy *n.* general lack of interest or enthusiasm

Approximate *adj.* almost but not completely accurate

Arbitrary *adj.* not seeming to be based on any plan or system

Arduous *adj.* difficult and tiring

Array *n.* an impressive display or range

Artificial selection *n.* the selective breeding of domesticated plants and animals to encourage the occurrence of desirable traits

Association *n.* a connection or link

Asthma *n.* a medical condition that causes difficulty in breathing

Asymptote *n.* (in mathematics) a line on the graph of a function, representing a value toward which the function may approach but does not reach; a line that continually approaches a given curve but does not meet it at any finite distance

Atherosclerosis *n.* a disease of the arteries characterized by the deposition of fatty material on their inner walls

Atmospheric *adj.* relating to the atmosphere of a planet

Atrophy *v.* gradual decline in effectiveness or vigor due to underuse or neglect

Audiologist *n.* medical professional who diagnoses and treats hearing and balance problems

Auditory *adj.* relating to hearing

Autoimmune disease *n.* condition in which the immune system mistakenly attacks the body

Baseline *n.* a starting point for comparisons

Biome *n.* a large, naturally occurring community of flora and fauna occupying a major habitat, e.g., forest or tundra

Biota *n.* the animal and plant life of a particular region, habitat, or geological period

Bohemian *adj.* an artistic and unconventional person

Bolster *v.* support or strengthen

Buffer *n.* to lessen the shock of; cushion

Calibrate *v.* compare the readings of an instrument with those of a standard

Calisthenics *n.* gymnastic exercise to achieve bodily fitness and grace of movement

Callus *n.* an area of thickened or hardened skin

Calorie *n.* a unit for measuring how much energy food will produce

Callousness *adj.* insensitive and cruel disregard for others

Canines *n.* pointed teeth next to the incisors with sharp surfaces for tearing food

Capacity *n.* the ability or power to do something

Capillary *n.* a microscopic blood vessel that penetrates the tissues and consists of a single layer of endothelial cells that allows exchange between the blood and interstitial fluid

Carelessness *n.* the act of not giving enough attention to avoid harm or mistakes; negligence

Cartilage *n.* a firm, flexible tissue that covers the ends of joints and forms structures, such as the external ear

Cells *n.* the smallest structural and functional unit of a living thing

Chagrin *n.* a feeling of disappointment or annoyance

Chemical *n.* any substance consisting of matter

Chemistry *n.* the branch of science concerned with the nature of substances and how they react with each other

Chronically *adv.* in a long-lasting or habitual and problematic way

Circadian rhythm *n.* a physiological cycle of about 24 hours that is present in all eukaryotic organisms and that persists even in the absence of external cues

Circulation *n.* the continuous movement of blood around the body

Clichéd *adj.* stereotypical or commonplace

Clinical *adj.* relating to the observation and treatment of patients

Coexistive *adv.* in a way that is together in harmony

Cohort *n.* group of individuals of the same age, from birth until all are dead

Coincide *v.* happen at the same time or place

Colic *n.* severe, often fluctuating pain in the abdomen caused by intestinal gas or an obstruction in the intestines and suffered especially by babies

Colon *n.* large intestine; the tubular portion of the vertebrate alimentary tract between the small intestine and the anus, functioning mainly in water absorption and the formation of feces

Compendium *n.* a collection of information about a subject

Complacency *n.* a feeling of smug or uncritical satisfaction with oneself or one's achievements

Component *n.* a part of a larger whole

Compound (1) *n.* a substance formed from two or more elements chemically united in fixed proportions (2) *v.* make something bad worse

Comprehensive *adj.* including or dealing with all or nearly all aspects of something

Comprise *v.* be made up of; consist of

Concentration *n.* the amount of a particular substance in a solution or mixture

Conclusive *adj.* decisive or convincing

Concoction *n.* a mixture of various ingredients or elements

Conditioning *n.* process of training or accustoming a person or animal to behave in a certain way or to accept certain circumstances

Conductive *adj.* having the property of conducting something (especially heat or electricity)

Confounded *v.* caused surprise or confusion, especially by acting against expectations

Conjecture *v.* to form an opinion based on incomplete information; to guess

Conscientious *adj.* careful and thorough in carrying out your work or duty

Conscious *adj.* aware of and responding to your surroundings; deliberate; intentional

Consecutive *adj.* following one after another in an unbroken sequence

Consequential *adj.* following as a result or effect

Consistent *adj.* always behaving in the same way; unchanging

Constraint *n.* a limitation or restriction

Contingency *n.* a plan made in case a particular thing happens

Contingent *adj.* dependent on

Contracting *v.* process of becoming shorter and tighter

Contrive *v.* plan or achieve something in a clever or skillful way

Conveyed *v.* communicated an idea or feeling

Convolutions *pl. n.* coils, twists or infoldings, especially one of many, in a thing that is complex and difficult to follow

Copacetic *adj.* (of a situation, mood, or relationship) being without problems; agreeable

Copulation *n.* sexual intercourse

Correlated *v.* placed things together so that one thing depends on another and vice versa

Correlation *n.* a situation in which one thing depends on another and vice versa

Counteract *v.* do something to reduce or prevent the bad effects of

Criticism *n.* expression of disapproval

Cues *n.* signals or prompts for action

Culmination *n.* the highest or climactic point of something

Data *n.* facts, figures, statistics, or other information

Daunting *adj.* seemingly difficult in anticipation

Debilitating *v.* severely weakening

Decrepit *adj.* worn out or ruined because of age or neglect

Deficiency *n.* a lack or shortage of something; a failing or shortcoming

Deficient *n.* not having enough of a particular quality or ingredient

Deficit *n.* the amount by which a total falls short of that required; shortage

Defecation *v.* process of expelling waste matter from the bowels

Deity *n.* a god or goddess

Deliberate *adj.* done on purpose; intentional and unhurried

Demise *n.* the end or failure of something

Depriving *v.* preventing from having or using something

Derived *v.* obtained something from a source; originated or developed from

Designed *v.* produced a design for; be intended for a purpose

Deteriorating *v.* becoming gradually worse; declining

Detrimental *adj.* causing harm or damage; harmful

Digestion *n.* process of digesting food; a being's ability to digest food

Diminish *v.* make or become smaller, weaker, or less

Discern *v.* recognize or be aware of; see or hear something with difficulty

Disjunct *adj.* disjoined and distinct from one another

Dispersed *v.* moved apart and went in different directions; thinned out and eventually disappeared

Disproportionate *adj.* too large or too small in comparison with something else

Dissipating *v.* disappearing or dispersing

Dissolve *v.* (of a solid) mix with a liquid and form a solution

Diversity *n.* the state of being varied; a range of different things

Dynamic *adj.* (of a process or system) constantly changing and developing

Dysfunction *n.* a state of inability to function properly

Earthship *n.* a type of passive solar shelter, made of both natural and upcycled materials, pioneered by architect Michael Reynolds

Ebb *v.* gradually become less or weaker

Eclectic *adj.* deriving ideas, style, or taste from a broad and diverse range of sources

Ecological *adj.* of or relating to the study of how animals and plants relate to one another and to their surroundings

Ecosystem *n.* all the plants and animals of a particular area considered in terms of how they interact with their environment

Efficient *adj.* working well, with no waste of money or effort

Ejaculation *v.* the process of ejecting semen from the body

Elaborate *v.* develop something in more detail

Elastic *adj.* able to go back to its normal shape after being stretched or squeezed; flexible

Elasticity *n.* ability of an object or material to resume its normal shape after being stretched or compressed

Electron *n.* a subatomic particle with a negative charge, found in all atoms

Eliminated *v.* completely removed or gotten rid of

Emaciated *adj.* abnormally thin and weak

Empathy *n.* the ability to understand and share the feelings of another

Emulate *v.* try to do as well or better than, usually by imitation

Epiphany *n.* a sudden and inspiring revelation

Equilibrium *n.* a state in which opposing forces are balanced; harmony

Encompass *v.* include a wide range of things; surround or cover

Enema *n.* a process in which liquid is injected into the rectum to clean it out

En masse *adv.* all together

Environment *n.* the surroundings in which a person, animal or plant lives and operates

Equilateral *adj.* having all its sides of the same length

Errant *adj.* traveling in search of adventure

Erratically *adj.* happening, moving, or acting in an uneven or irregular way

Essential *adj.* absolutely necessary

Evince *v.* reveal the presence of

Evolutionarily *adv.* in a way that relates to evolution or gradual development

Evolve *v.* develop and change over many generations by the process of evolution

Exacerbated *v.* made something that is already bad worse

Excitation *n.* the application of energy to a particle, object, or physical system

Excrete *v.* pass waste material from the body

Exertion *n.* physical or mental effort

Exfoliated *v.* shed from a surface in scales or layers

Exhibit *v.* show a particular quality

Exorbitant *adj.* unreasonably high

Extract *v.* separate out a substance by a special method; remove with care or effort

Fatigue *n.* great tiredness

Fauna *n.* the animals of a particular region or period

Feasible *adj.* able to be done easily; possible

Feedback *n.* information about reactions to something, used as a basis for improvement

Fertilization *v.* the process of introducing sperm or pollen into an egg or plant so that a new individual develops

Flora *n.* the plants of a particular region or period

Foraging *v.* (of a person or animal) searching widely for food or provisions

Foray *n.* an organized group going in search of fungi

Fortitude *n.* courage or strength when facing pain or trouble

Frequency *n.* (1) the rate at which something happens; (2) the number of cycles per second of a sound, light, or radio wave; a particular waveband at which radio waves are transmitted

Function *n.* (1) a purpose or natural activity of a person or thing; (2) (in math) a quantity whose value depends on the varying values of others

Fungus *n.* an organism, such as a mushroom, that has no leaves or flowers and grows on plants or decaying vegetable matter and reproduces by spores

Furtive *adj.* secretly trying to avoid being noticed

Genetic *adj.* relating to genes or to the field of genetics

Genetics *pl. n.* the study of the way characteristics are passed from one generation to another

Genetic modification *n.* the process of altering the genetic makeup of an organism to produce a desired characteristic

Genitalia *n.* male or female reproductive parts, whether internal or external; the genitals

Genome *n.* the complete set of genetic material of an organism

Gullible *adj.* easily believing what people tell you

Habitat *n.* the natural home or environment of a plant or animal

Hemorrhoid *n.* a swollen vein in the region of the anus

Hernia *n.* a condition in which part of an organ or fatty tissue pushes through the wall of the cavity containing it

Hindrance *n.* a thing that provides resistance, delay, or obstruction to something or someone

Holistic *adj.* characterized by comprehension of the parts of something as intimately interconnected and explicable only by reference to the whole

Hormone *n.* in multicellular organisms, one of many types of circulating chemical signals that are formed in specialized cells, travel in body fluids, and act on specific target cells to change their functioning

Humility *n.* the quality of having a modest opinion of your own importance

Hygiene *n.* the practice of keeping yourself and your surroundings clean in order to prevent illness and disease

Hygienically *adv.* free from pathogenic elements or environments; sanitary

Hypothermia *n.* a condition in which the body loses heat faster than it can produce heat, causing a dangerously low body temperature

Idiosyncratic *adj.* in a distinctive or peculiar way; relating to a person's particular way of behaving or thinking

Ignorance *n.* lack of knowledge or information

Immerse *v.* to involve oneself deeply in a particular interest or activity

Immune system *n.* complex system of cells, tissues, and organs and the substances they make that helps the body to fight infections and diseases

Immunity *n.* the body's ability to resist a particular infection

Impending *adj.* be about to happen; imminent

Inadvertently *adv.* unintentionally

Inauspicious *adj.* not conducive to success; unpromising

Incentive *n.* something that motivates, encourages, or influences one to do something

Incessantly *adj.* constantly; without interruption

Incongruity *n.* the state of being out of place; inappropriate

Incorporated *v.* included something as part of a whole; integrated

Incrementally *adv.* in regular increases, additions, or stages

Indifference *n.* lack of interest, concern, or sympathy

Indigenous *adj.* belonging to a place; native

Induce *v.* bring about or cause

Inevitably *adv.* unavoidably

Infancy *n.* the early stage in the development or growth of something; the state or period of babyhood

Inference *n.* a conclusion reached on the basis of evidence and reasoning; deduction

Infirmity *n.* physical or mental weakness

Inflammation *n.* a localized physical condition in which an area of the body becomes swollen, red, hot, and often painful, especially as a reaction to injury or infection

Inflammatory bowel disease *n.* a term for conditions characterized by chronic inflammation of the gastrointestinal tract

Influx *n.* the arrival or entry of large numbers of things

Ingest *v.* take food, drink, or other substances into the body by swallowing or absorbing them

Ingrained *adj.* firmly established; deeply embedded

Innards *pl. n.* internal organs

Innate *adj.* natural or inborn

Integration *n.* the action or process of combining with something to make a whole; bringing into equal participation

Integrative *adj.* serving or intending to unify separate things

Integrity *n.* the quality of being honest, fair, and good

Intermittent *adj.* stopping and starting at irregular intervals

Intestinal *adj.* relating to or affecting the long tube running from the stomach to the anus

Intrinsic *adj.* forming part of the fundamental nature of something

Invasive *adj.* involving the introduction of instruments or other objects into the body

Involuntarily *adv.* without will or conscious control

Iteration *n.* the repetition of a process or utterance

Jaded *adj.* tired, bored, or lacking enthusiasm, typically after having too much of something

Lateral *adj.* of, at, toward, or from the side or sides

Liability *n.* a person or thing whose presence or behavior is likely to cause embarrassment or put one at a disadvantage

Life expectancy *n.* the predicted average length of life

Ligament *n.* a band of connective tissue connecting bone to bone, often serving to hold together a joint

LSD *n.* lysergic acid diethylamide, a drug that causes hallucinations

Macroscopic *adj.* large enough to be seen without a microscope

Maiming *v.* inflicting a permanent injury on

Mammalian *adj.* of or relating to mammals, which are warm-blooded animals that have body hair or fur, produce milk, and give birth to live young

Masochist *n.* a person who enjoys painful or tedious activities

Matter *n.* a physical substance or material; anything that takes up space and has mass

Melatonin *n.* a hormone secreted by the pineal gland that regulates body functions related to seasonal day length

Membrane *n.* a skin-like tissue that connects, covers, or lines cells or parts of the body

Mentally *adv.* in a manner relating to the mind

Metabolic *adj.* of or relating to the process by which food is used for the growth of tissue or the production of energy

Metabolic momentum *n.* the tendency of metabolism to continue in one direction or another, even after precursory stimuli (like the intake of food) has ceased

Metabolite *n.* substance formed in or necessary for metabolism

Meticulous *adj.* very careful and precise

Microbe *n.* a microorganism; very small living thing

Microbial *adj.* of or relating to microbes

Microbiome *n.* all of the microorganisms in a given environment

Microscopic *adj.* so small as to be visible only through a microscope

Mineral *n.* an inorganic substance needed by the body for good health

Misconstruing *v.* interpreting something wrongly (especially words or actions)

Moderate *adj.* average in amount, strength, or degree

Moderation *n.* the avoidance of extremes, in action or opinion

Molar *n.* a grinding tooth, at the back of the mouth

Molecule *n.* a group of atoms forming the smallest unit into which a substance may be divided

Montessori *n.* a system of education for young children that seeks to develop natural interests and activities rather than formal education

Mortality *n.* death

Mundane *adj.* lacking interest or excitement

Musculoskeletal *adj.* relating to or denoting the musculature and skeleton together

Myriad *n.* a countless or very great number

Naturopathic *adj.* of or relating to naturopathy, a form of healthcare that combines modern treatment with traditional methods and centers on the body's capacity to heal itself

Nested *v.* fit an object inside a larger one

Neurotransmitter *n.* a chemical substance released from a nerve fiber and bringing about the transfer of an impulse to another nerve, muscle, etc.

Niche *n.* the match of a species to specific ecological environment, describing how an organism or population responds to the distribution of resources and competitors and how it in turn alters those same factors

Nomadic *adj.* having the natural inclination to wander with no fixed habitation

Noni *n.* any of various evergreen trees or shrubs of the Madder family, native to the South Pacific; various medicinal preparations are made from their leaves, roots, and fruit

Novel *adj.* new, in an interesting or unusual way

Nutriment *n.* nourishment

Nutrition *n.* the process of providing or obtaining the food necessary for health and growth

Obligatory *adj.* required by a law, rule, or custom; compulsory

Olfactory *adj.* relating to the sense of smell

Optimal *adj.* best or most favorable

Organism *n.* an individual animal, plant, or life-form

Orientation *n.* a position in relation to something else

Orthodox *adj.* in keeping with generally accepted beliefs; normal

Osteopath *n.* a licensed physician who aims to improve a patient's overall health and wellness by treating the whole person, not just a condition or disease they have

Overexert *v.* engage in too much or too strenuous exertion

Overt *adj.* done or shown openly

Palatable *adj.* pleasant to taste; acceptable

Parameter *n.* a thing that decides or limits the way in which something else can be done

Particle *n.* a minute piece of matter

Pathogenic *adj.* (of a bacteria, virus, or other microorganism) disease-causing

Penitence *n.* the action of feeling or showing sorrow and regret for having done wrong; repentance

Perceive *v.* become conscious or aware of something through the senses; come to realize or understand

Permeate *v.* spread throughout

Perpetually *adv.* in a way that is never ending or changing; so frequent as to seem continual

Perpetuate *v.* cause something to continue indefinitely

Persistent *adj.* continuing or recurring over a long period

Perspective *n.* a particular attitude toward or way of regarding something; point of view

Pheromone *n.* a small, volatile chemical substance produced and released into the environment by a plant, animal, or fungi, which affects the behavior or physiology of nearby organisms, especially those of the same species

Physically *adv.* of or relating to the body rather than the mind; relating to things that may be seen, heard, or felt

Physical therapy *n.* the treatment of disease or injury by physical methods such as massage, heat treatment, and exercise

Physiological *adj.* of or relating to the scientific study of the way in which living things function

Pinnacle *n.* the most successful or highest point

Placebo *n.* a substance with no healing effect, given to some participants in a drug trial for comparison

Plethora *n.* an excessive amount or number of something

Pollen *n.* a powder produced by the male part of a flower, which is carried by bees, the wind, etc., and can fertilize other flowers; the male gametophyte of seed plants

Posterior *adj.* pertaining to the rear, or tail end, of a bilaterally symmetrical animal; at or near the rear

Preclusion *n.* something that prevents or makes impossible; the act of preventing something or making it impossible

Predilection *n.* a preference or special liking for something; a bias in favor of something

Preliminary *adj.* taking place before a main action or event

Prematurely *adv.* before the proper time

Premolar *n.* a tooth situated between the canine and the molar teeth; an adult human usually has eight, two in each jaw on each side

Primate *n.* an order of mammals distinguishable by their having hands, feet similar to hands, and forward-facing eyes; this group includes tarsiers, lemurs, lorises, monkeys, apes, and humans

Primitive *adj.* relating to, denoting, or preserving the character of an early stage in the evolutionary or historical development of something

Proboscis *n.* an elongated sucking mouthpart that is typically tubular and flexible

Proclivity *n.* a tendency to do something regularly

Proficient *adj.* competent; skilled

Profuse *adj.* produced or appearing in large quantities

Promote *v.* help something to happen

Propensity *n.* a tendency to behave in a particular way

Proportion *n.* the relationship of one thing to another in terms or quantity or size

Prostate *n.* a gland in male mammals that produces the fluid part of semen

Protruding *adj.* sticking out from a surface; jutting

Protrusion *n.* something that protrudes; a protuberance

Psoriasis *n.* a skin disease marked by red, itchy, scaly patches

Psychosomatic *adj.* a physical response induced by the mind, through belief, stress, or anxiety

Qualm *n.* an uneasy feeling of doubt, worry, or fear, especially about one's own conduct; misgiving

Quantifying *v.* expressing or measuring the quantity of

Rampant *adj.* flourishing or spreading unchecked (especially of something unpleasant or unwelcome)

Rate *n.* a measure, quantity or frequency measured against another; the speed of something

Recognizing *v.* accepting something as genuine, legal, or valid

Reconciling *v.* making or showing to be compatible; causing to exist in harmony

Recuperate *v.* recover from illness or exertion

Recuperative *adj.* having the effect of restoring health or strength

Recurring *v.* happening again or repeatedly

Reduce *v.* make or become less

Redundantly *adv.* to do in such a way as to make the action being done no longer necessary or superfluous

Relinquishing *v.* voluntarily ceasing to keep or claim; giving up

Replenish *v.* fill up a supply again after using some of it; restock

Representation *n.* expression or designation by some symbol, image, model, etc., of something

Reproach *n.* an expression of disapproval or disappointment

Resilient *adj.* able to withstand or recover quickly from difficult conditions

Respiration *n.* the action of breathing

Resurgence *n.* an increase after a period of little activity or occurrence

Retracting *v.* pulling back; drawing something back

Reveled in *v.* enjoyed something very much

Rickets *n.* the softening and weakening of bones in children, usually in response to extreme and prolonged vitamin D deficiency

Rupture *v.* break or burst suddenly

Saliva *n.* a watery liquid in the mouth produced by glands that helps to lubricate food, adhere together chewed pieces, and begin the process of chemical digestion

Scarce *adj.* (of a resource) only available in small quantities that do not meet demand; in short supply

Scoliosis *n.* abnormal lateral (sideways) curvature of the spine

Secrete *v.* (of a cell, gland, or organ) discharge of a substance synthesized for a particular function in the organism or for excretion

Secretion *n.* a substance that has been secreted

Sequential *adj.* following in a logical order or sequence

Serotonin *n.* a compound secreted by the central nervous system and taken up by blood platelets, which constricts the blood vessels and acts as a neurotransmitter to modulate mood, cognition, reward, learning, memory, and numerous other physiological processes

Spectrum *n.* used to classify something in terms of its position on a scale between two extreme or opposite points

Speed wobble *v.* quick oscillation of the steerable wheels leading to increasing full-vehicle yaw oscillations and loss of control, which may occur on any vehicle with a single steering pivot point and a sufficient amount of freedom of the steered wheel, such as a motorcycle, skateboard, bicycle, or tricycle-style landing gear on some aircraft

Sperm *n.* (aka spermatazoan) the male sex cell of an animal, which fertilizes the egg

Spore *n.* a tiny reproductive cell produced by fungi and many plants

Spotter *n.* someone who is available to assist in a lift or exercise if needed

Sterile *adj.* free from bacteria or other living microorganisms; thoroughly clean

Sternum *n.* the breastbone

Steroid *n.* a class of internal signaling molecule, found in plants, animals, and fungi

Stimulation *n.* the action of arousing interest, enthusiasm, or excitement

Stimuli *pl. n.* some things that stimulate

Stimulus *n.* something that stimulates

Stint *n.* a fixed or allotted period of work

Strenuous *adj.* needing or using a lot of effort or exertion

Structure *n.* an object constructed from several parts

Structured *v.* put parts together to form a whole

Stunted *v.* prevented from growing or developing properly

Subconscious *adj.* concerning the part of the mind that you are not aware of but that influences your thoughts and feelings

Subsequent *adj.* coming after something; following

Subtle *adj.* (especially of a change or distinction) so delicate or precise as to be difficult to describe or analyze

Successive *adj.* following one another or following others; sequential

Succinct *adj.* briefly and clearly expressed

Supplement *n.* a thing added to something else to improve or complete it

Suppress *v.* forcibly put an end to; prevent from acting or developing

Surreal *adj.* strange and having the qualities of a dream

Susceptible *adj.* likely to be influenced or harmed by; vulnerable to

Sustain *v.* (1) keep something going over time or continuously; (2) experience something unpleasant

Symbiotic *adj.* of or relating to an ecological relationship between organisms of two different species that live together in direct contact

Symmetry *n.* the exact match in size or shape between two halves, parts, or sides of something

Tangible *adj.* able to be perceived by touch; real

Temperate *adj.* (of a region or climate) having mild temperatures

Tenacity *n.* the quality or fact of being very determined or persistent; determination

Tendon *n.* a strong band or cord of tissue attaching a muscle to a bone

Testosterone *n.* a sex hormone that stimulates the development of male physical characteristics and plays many other important roles in the body; in men it is thought to regulate libido (sex drive), bone mass, fat distribution, muscle mass and strength, and the production of red blood cells and sperm

Toxic *adj.* poisonous; relating to or caused by poison

Trait *n.* a distinguishing quality or characteristic; any detectable variation in a genetic character

Trigger *n.* an event that causes something to happen or exist

Trucks *pl. n.* (on a skateboard) the axle component, which couples the deck to the wheels

Turmeric *n.* an aromatic, bright-yellow powder obtained from a plant in the ginger family and used in Asian cooking

Ultimately *adv.* in the end; finally

Unorthodox *adj.* different from what is usual, traditional, or accepted

Uptake *v.* the taking in or absorption of a substance by a living organism or bodily organ

Uterine *adj.* of or relating to the uterus or womb

Variable *n.* an element, feature, or factor that is liable to vary or change

Variation *n.* (1) a change or slight difference in condition, amount, or level; (2) a different or distinct form or version

Vegetation *n.* plants

Vegetative *adj.* of or relating to vegetation

Vertebrate *n.* an animal having a backbone (i.e., fish, mammal, bird, reptile, or amphibian)

Vigor *n.* (1) physical strength and good health; (2) effort, energy, and enthusiasm

Visual *adj.* relating to seeing or sight

Vividly *adv.* in a way that produces powerful feelings or strong, clear images in the mind

Volition *n.* a being's will or power of independent action

Voraciously *adv.* excessively eagerly; insatiably

Wane *v.* become smaller or weaker

Wax *v.* become larger or stronger

RECOMMENDED READING

These are books that have been especially influential in the formation of my personal beliefs, my perception of the universe, and my sense of my own body, some of which were mentioned within the text.

The Celestine Prophecy by James Redfield © 1997

The Life You Were Born to Live by Dan Millman © 1993

Sound Mind, Sound Body by Dr. Kenneth R. Pelletier © 1995

Rich Dad, Poor Dad by Robert Kiyosaki and Sharon Lechter © 1997

Perfect Health: the Complete Mind/Body Guide by Deepak Chopra © 1991

The Secrets of Female Sexuality by David Shade © 2009

Be Here Now by Ram Dass © 1971

REFERENCES

Alcock, John. *Animal Behavior: An Evolutionary Approach.* 8th edition. Chapter 14: "The Evolution of Human Behavior," 479–511. Sunderland, MA: Sinauer Associates, 2005.

Allen, John S., Susan C. Anton, and Craig Stanford. *Exploring Biological Anthropology: The Essentials.* Chapter 10: "Early Hominids and Australopithecus," 242–75. Upper Saddle River, NJ: Pearson Education, 2008.

Arulselvan, P., M. T. Fard, W. S. Tan, S. Gothai, S. Fakurazi, M. E. Norhaizan, and S. S. Kumar. "Role of Antioxidants and Natural Products in Inflammation." *Oxidative Medicine and Cellular Longevity* 2016 (2016), 5276130. https://doi.org/10.1155/2016/5276130.

Burke, C. A. "Mindfulness-Based Approaches with Children and Adolescents: A Preliminary Review of Current Research in an Emergent Field." *Journal of Child and Family Studies* 19 (2010), 133–44.

Friedman P. K., and I. B. Lamster. "Tooth Loss as a Predictor of Shortened Longevity: Exploring the Hypothesis." *Periodontology 2000* 71, no. 1 (October 2016): 142–52. https://doi.org/10.1111/prd.12128.

Gilbert, Jack, Martin J. Blaser, J. Gregory Caporaso, Janet Jansson, Susan V. Lynch, and Rob Knight. "Current Understanding of the Human Microbiome." *Nature Medicine* 24, no. 4 (April 10, 2018): 392–400.

J. Fröhlich-Nowoisky, et al. "High Diversity of Fungi in Air Particulate Matter." *PNAS* 106, no. 31 (July 17, 2009), 12814–12819. https://doi.org/10.1073/pnas.0811003106.

Lautenbacher, S., J. Peters, M. Heesen, et al. "Age Changes in Pain Perception: A Systematic-Review and Meta-Analysis of Age Effects on Pain and Tolerance Thresholds." *Neuroscience and Biobehavioral Reviews* 75 (April 2017): 104–13. https://doi.org/10.1016/j.neubiorev.2017.01.039.

Ober, Clinton, Stephen T. Sinatra, and Martin Zucker. *Earthing: The Most Important Health Discovery Ever?* Laguna Beach, CA: Basic Health Publications, 2010.

"Preamble to the Constitution of WHO as Adopted by the International Health Conference, New York, 19 June–22 July 1946; Signed on 22 July 1946 by the Representatives of 61 States, and Entered into Force on 7 April 1948." Official Records of WHO, no. 2: 100.

Reece, Jane B., and Neil A. Campbell. *Campbell Biology*. Boston: Benjamin Cummings/Pearson, 2011.

Russell, J. B., and New York State College of Agriculture and Life Sciences. *Rumen Microbiology and Its Role in Ruminant Nutrition*. Ithaca, NY: Department of Microbiology, Cornell University, 2002.

Schmale, J., et al. "Collocated Observations of Cloud Condensation Nuclei, Particle Size Distributions, and Chemical Composition." *Scientific Data* 4 (2017): 170003. https://doi.org/10.1038/sdata.2017.3.